THE BELLY OFF! DIET™

ATTACK THE FAT THAT MATTERS MOST

By Jeff Csatari
and the editors of Men'sHealth

RODALE

The Belly Off! Diet is a registered trademark of Rodale Inc.

Men's Health is a registered trademark of Rodale Inc.

Rodale books may be purchased for business or promotional use or for special sales. For information, please write to:

Special Markets Department, Rodale Inc., 733 Third Avenue, New York, NY 10017

Printed in the United States of America

Rodale Inc. makes every effort to use acid-free ♾, recycled paper ♻.

Cover and interior photographs by © Thomas MacDonald/Rodale Images

Book design by Andrezej Janerka

Library of Congress Cataloging-in-Publication Data on file with the publisher.

ISBN 13: 978–1–60529–821–4

ISBN 10: 1–60529–821–2

Distributed to the trade by Macmillan

2 4 6 8 10 9 7 5 3 1   hardcover

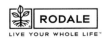

RODALE
LIVE YOUR WHOLE LIFE™

We inspire and enable people to improve their lives and the world around them
For more of our products visit **rodalestore.com** or call 800-848-4735

Dedicated to the men in the Belly Off! Club
who generously shared their stories about losing weight
and improving their health to inspire others to do the same.

"It's a lot harder to rationalize a double cheeseburger if you know you'll have a black-and-white record of it."

—Belly Off! Club member DAVE KAHN

on keeping a food journal for motivation

CONTENTS

PART IV
MAKING THE BELLY OFF! DIET
WORK FOR YOU

ACKNOWLEDGMENTS

First, let me raise a protein shake to toast the men who have opened up their lives and shared their weight-loss stories through the Belly Off! Club department in *Men's Health*. Without your inspiring examples, *The Belly Off! Diet* and its online companion at menshealth.com/bellyoff would not exist.

My deepest gratitude goes to those who gave me the opportunity to work on this book: the Rodale family, who continue to inspire people to live greener and healthier lives, to Steve Murphy, the president and CEO of Rodale Inc., for his dedication to editorial excellence and our mission to serve our readers; and David Zinczenko, for his longtime support and encouragement, and his tireless efforts on behalf of the *Men's Health* brand.

Many thanks to all those who shepherded this project and its many moving parts through to completion, especially my editor, Courtney Conroy; *Men's Health* brand editor Bill Stump; Joe Heroun and George Karabotsos, who designed the cover; book designer Andrezej Janerka; model and trainer David Jack; Joanna Williams, Marc Sirinsky, Susan Eugster, and Lois Hazel; and the team at menshealth.com who give the Belly Off! Club a robust presence on the Web, especially Sean Nolan, Kevin Donahue, and Greg Presto.

To generous colleagues and friends who've taught me tons of useful stuff along the way, including Mark Bricklin, William Butterworth IV, Adam Campbell, Matt Marion, Peter Moore, Hugh O'Neill, Steve Perrine, Bill Phillips, Bill Stieg, and Jim Thornton, and all the talented editors, designers, photo editors, and writers with whom I've shared time in the trenches at *Men's Health* and *Best Life* magazines.

My family—Joseph, Susan, Joe, and Wendy—and the rest of the Hungarian Hoedown crowd at LBI.

And to my best friend, Kathy, and our daughters, Katelyn, Lydia, and Sophia, who bring me such tremendous joy every day. Thank you for putting up with the late nights and the mess on the dining room table.

FOREWORD

Let's say you run into a buddy of yours whom you haven't seen in a while. He has lost 50 pounds, looks about 10 years younger, and is bursting with energy that you wouldn't mind having. Wouldn't you be just a little bit curious to know how he did it?

We would. And that's sort of how this book came about. You see, for the past 8 years, in each issue of *Men's Health* magazine, we've published a simple success story like that about one man's struggle to lose weight and shape up. We call it The Belly Off! Club, and on this page we chronicle his transformation from fat man to fit man.

Month in and month out, The Belly Off! Club is one of the most-read sections of the magazine, and it is extremely popular on our Web site, menshealth.com, as well. In fact, within a month of launching Belly Off! on the Web site, the club surpassed 20,000 members. Today, more than 300,000 men in the Belly Off! Club have lost nearly 2 million pounds! Curious to know just how they did it—and to inform his own weight-loss efforts—author Jeff Csatari pored through the old research files from the articles of the 80-plus men who've graced our Belly Off! Club page since 2001 and reviewed more case histories from the Web site. He quickly noticed an emerging pattern. Our big belly losers all used the same handful of techniques to drop 20, 60, 90, even more than 150 pounds!

The *Men's Health* Belly Off! Diet is based on those tips and techniques and the groundbreaking science that supports them. And it is your best tool for finally winning your battle with weight and taking off that belly of yours for good. This plan isn't about a special food or counting calories or fancy fitness gadgets. It's about real men doing old-school exercise at home. It's about eating really good food—guy food that tastes great, fills you up, and satisfies your hunger so you won't overeat. Part of the magic of this book is that it's based in reality, not restriction; and these myriad get-back-in-shape solutions take into account your ever-changing goals and circumstances—so you always have ways to get your best body ever and keep it for life.

Most important, if you are overweight, *The Belly Off! Diet* will help you to significantly improve your health and lower your risk for dangers like diabetes and heart disease. That's why I am proud of this *Men's Health* book and believe it is so important for men today. Being overweight has just surpassed smoking as the leading cause of premature heart attacks in this country. Let's fight this trend one belly at a time.

Join the Belly Off! Club and start attacking the fat that matters most.

DAVID ZINCZENKO
Editor-in-Chief, *Men's Health*
December 15, 2008

PART I

Join the Belly Off! Club

1

THE SECRETS OF BELLY OFF! SUCCESS

Your Plan to Finally Lose That Gut Starts Here

YOU MAY HAVE PICKED UP THIS BOOK because you are feeling a bit flabbier than you felt a few years ago and you want to get back in shape. Some of you may have struggled with your weight for years and you are understandably concerned about your health. Whatever your personal weight and fitness situation, the Belly Off! Diet will help you. That's a promise. I've seen it work for others. I've felt it myself.

When I started researching this book, I wasn't what you might call *overweight,* but I certainly wasn't cover-model material for *Men's Health* magazine, where I work—even if they *could* Photoshop Matthew McConaughey's chiseled features over mine.

I would suck wind when I played basketball at noon

with the guys on staff. And when I reluctantly took off my shirt at the community pool, my middle oozed over my waistband like a roll of Coney Island taffy. My younger brother Joe, for the first time in our lives, could bench-press more than me. *Ouch.*

I had turned into a soft-bodied, middle-aged suburban dad eating my kids' leftover Happy Meals.

Then one day, I got a wake-up call. A buddy phoned to tell me that a friend had died of a massive heart attack—at age 49. Coincidentally, 2 days later, the nation learned about the passing of *Meet the Press* moderator Tim Russert—at age 58. Both men died so terribly young. Tragic happenings like this tend to make you focus on the things that really should always be on top of your mind—things like your family, your purpose in life, and your health. I started thinking, as I'm sure a lot of guys did: *I'm not invincible. That could happen to me. It is high time that I start taking better care of myself.*

Most of us should. Today, two-thirds of Americans have excess body fat, and nearly a third can be classified as full-blown obese. It's no secret that being overweight can dramatically increase your risk of diabetes, high blood pressure, heart disease, gallbladder disease, sleep apnea, and cancer. But new research in 2008 found that obesity has now overtaken smoking as the leading cause of premature heart attacks, according to a report in the *Journal of the American College of Cardiology*. Researchers studying more than 111,000 heart attack patients found that while the average age of a first heart attack was 74.6 years in the leanest patients, it was 58.7 years in the most obese.

"The leading theory in cardiology right now is that the fat tissue is actually producing factors that precipitate heart attacks," says study author Peter McCullough, MD, a cardiologist and chief of nutrition and prevention medicine at William Beaumont Hospital in Royal Oak, Michigan. Dr. McCullough says that a person with a body mass index of more than 40 can expect a heart attack 12 years earlier than a person with a BMI of 25 to 30. (For an explanation of body mass index, see page 20.)

After the death of my friend, I considered my own family's health history—high blood pressure, heart attacks, diabetes, and cancer. It's all there. It may be there in your family, too. If you don't know, ask.

Well, it was motivation enough for me.

So, I laced up my running shoes and began sweating every day. I cut the Oreos and chocolate cake from my diet, gave away my case of Sierra Nevada Pale Ale to a thirsty friend, and picked up my dumbbells again.

It wasn't easy. Changing long-practiced eating habits never is. And finding the time to exercise, well, you know it's never easy. But in less than 2 weeks, my sore body started to feel pretty good! I was already lighter by 6 pounds, and I didn't feel like hurling in the middle of my runs. Some of the quickest successes come in the beginning of a disciplined workout/diet regimen, mine included. In 3 weeks, I had dropped 14 pounds. I was running faster, sleeping better, and feeling energized and happier.

REAL-WORLD RESULTS

All that may sound like the stuff of late-night infomercials, but, actually, my 14 pounds is *nothing* compared to the accomplishments of the men you'll meet in this book. That's where you should look for motivation. The Belly Off! Diet is based on the real-world examples of men whose stories have been chronicled in the Belly Off! Club column in *Men's Health* magazine over the past 8 years, plus the weight-loss strategies of some of the 300,000 other men who've signed up for the *Men's Health* Belly Off! Club on our Web site, www.menshealth.com/bellyoff. All told, over the years since the Belly Off! Club began, men have lost nearly 2 million pounds. More important, they've dramatically improved their health and reduced their risk for life-threatening diseases.

Draw inspiration from guys like Brandon Watford of Bonifay, Florida, whose physician recommended a gastric bypass because his life was in jeopardy. At 374 pounds, Watford would get winded climbing just a few steps. But he refused the surgery, and he committed

IT WORKS FOR ME

"Even if you don't feel like working out, tell yourself you'll do at least 10 minutes. When those minutes are up, your endorphins will be pumping, and it'll be easier to continue."

—Brian Bray, Gainesville, FL, who lost 130 pounds

himself to making lifestyle changes—small ones at first. Nonetheless, simple changes to his diet and a regular exercise plan helped him cut his weight nearly in half. "I've added years back to my life," he says.

Or consider Dan Sizelove, who topped 290 pounds as a result of poor food choices and late-night partying. The former college football player felt a void in his life, but it certainly wasn't in his belly. He missed being active. So he started running and biking, then added weight training. He ditched the chips and made an effort to eat more protein, which helped him shed 80 pounds. His energy level skyrocketed. "I don't need coffee to wake up anymore," he says.

Then there's Tony Fedora who used the Belly Off! Club cardio and bodyweight exercises at www. menshealth.com/bellyoff to lose more than 50 pounds in just 3 months. "I started using the warehouse where I work as a makeshift gym," he says. "I do pullups off the forklift and use 5-gallon bottles of water from the water machines to do deadlifts. And when I'm the last one to leave, I'll do walking lunges over to the light switch, which is a football field away."

This book is filled with examples of men like these guys, who share their weight-loss strategies and personal tips from their journey to better health.

THE SIX SECRETS OF WEIGHT LOSS

How did so many men lose so many pounds? We were curious to know exactly how, too, so we dusted off the dog-eared copies of *Men's Health* going back to January 2001, all 80-something issues, and reread every Belly Off! Club story. We pulled out the research files for those articles and pored through each report, searching for the common strategies that have helped all of these men shed their big bellies. Not only were we once again inspired by their stories, but we found something surprising: We noticed the same six weight-loss techniques over and over again. Most men who appeared in the *Men's Health* Belly Off! Club column shared the same simple strategies, whether they lost 10 pounds, 60 pounds, 100, or even 150 pounds! Check it out:

- **96 percent** cut way back on foods with refined flour and added sugars like those found in juices, sodas, white bread, rice, cookies, and cakes, substituting more fruits, vegetables, and fiber-rich whole grains.

- **93 percent** say they now eat more lean protein and healthy fats.

- **75 percent** reported eating more often—four to six times a day—spacing their calories out to keep their metabolisms revving high.

- **90 percent** do muscle-building resistance exercises three or more times a week.

- **88 percent** do cardio exercises like running, biking, swimming, playing tennis or basketball, and practicing martial arts.

- **85 percent** said that portion control is a crucial part of their weight-loss strategy.

FAT FACT

11

Number of miles you would have to run to burn off the 1,534 calories in a large cheeseburger and french fries.

If the above techniques can work so well for these guys (and their brethren at www.menshealth.com/bellyoff), do you think they might do the trick for you? We do. Because every one of those real-world, regular-guy strategies is backed by the latest research on exercise, nutrition, and weight loss. They work in the lab. They work at home.

WHAT TO EXPECT

This book is built upon those six core strategies that have helped our guys lose weight fast and keep it off. Make them a part of your daily routine and you will lose significant pounds in 4 weeks and start seeing results within the first 5 days. That's no vacant promise. This program will work because it's based on science—and, frankly, it's logical. You and I know that

there is no magic bullet for sustainable weight loss. No
single food. No single exercise. No machine or pill or
revolutionary diet of denial that's going to do your work
for you. To lose weight you must make several important lifestyle changes and stick with them. That's what
this plan is about—making them easy to follow and
easy to maintain. Here's what you can expect from the
Belly Off! Diet over the next 4 weeks:

- **You won't feel hungry.** In fact, you'll eat more frequently than you do now, four to six times a day.

- **Your meals will be guy foods that you love**—steak,
  eggs, chicken, meatloaf, fish, chili, tacos, and
  pizza. We at *Men's Health* firmly believe that
  most of us cannot go long periods without
  certain staples of male cuisine and that sacrificing these joys is a sure way to doom any diet.

- **You won't have to count calories or grams of fat.** If
  you get about a third of your calories from protein
  (don't worry; you won't need math to figure it out),
  eat a little satisfying fat, and pack fiber into every
  meal, you'll automatically eat fewer junk carbs—
  carbs that cause dangerous belly fat to expand.
  Healthier eating will take care of itself. In a 2007
  study, Purdue University researchers found that
  people who ate this way lost more weight faster
  than those who didn't eat much protein.

- **You'll eat lots of vegetables.** As much as you want
  of those rich in fiber. Why? Because they are low
  in calories, high in volume due to their water
  content, and jam-packed with healthy nutrients.

- **You'll learn a simple eating strategy that can actually deactivate the gene** that's responsible for
  producing dangerous blood fats called triglycerides that play a role in fat storage in the body.

- **You'll snack on nuts, cheese, and fruit.**

- **You'll drink lots of water**—or milk, tea, and coffee,
  if you wish—but you'll knock off the beer, hard

liquor, and sugary drinks. We're not saying that you can never have these again. Just not now. Not until you make some significant progress. Banning alcoholic drinks will give you a tremendous head start.

■ **You'll exercise three to six times a week,** but never for more than 45 minutes and you won't have to go to a gym if you don't care to.

■ **You'll do some interval training**—short bursts of intense exercise followed by rest paces—because new research shows that interval training triggers your cells to burn belly fat *first*.

■ **You'll use a workout strategy developed by weight-loss researchers** at the University of Connecticut that can actually cancel out the effects of a high-calorie meal!

And you'll lose weight fast, mostly from your belly region—as much as 8 to 10 pounds and an inch from your waist in the first 2 weeks. But even more important, you'll reap benefits that you can't see—benefits that may save your life. This program will significantly reduce your risk of developing prediabetes; cardiovascular disease, the biggest killer of guys like us; and cancers of the stomach, colon, and prostate.

THE BELLY OFF! DIET AND FITNESS PLAN

The nuts and bolts of the program are:

1. **A 7-Day Quick-Start** that'll familiarize you with the principal techniques and deliver fast results
2. **The Bodyweight 100 no-gear workout series** that doesn't require a huge commitment of time or a pricey membership to a gym (you can do these exercises at home)
3. **Real Meals**—easy recipes for guy foods that won't go to your gut

The 7-Day Quick-Start is a day-by-day schedule of how to eat and how to exercise. We'll tell you exactly what to do. No thinking. Just follow the plan and you'll feel it working. You'll start each day with the Belly Off! Diet 2-Minute Drill—eight calisthenics designed to spark your metabolism. Do them in your boxer shorts. Then you'll eat a satisfying breakfast. Do these two things and you'll set yourself up for all-day fat burning. The 7-Day Quick-Start includes a shopping list of everything you need to follow the meal plan for 7 days. We'll get you out of the grocery store in under an hour, and you'll eat healthily for a week. The 7-Day Quick-Start is crucial because it establishes a pattern of healthy habits that will soon become just a natural part of your life.

The Bodyweight 100 series is a simple circuit of exercises that uses only your bodyweight for resistance, so you can do them anywhere—even in a hotel room on a business trip. No gear needed. No excuses for not doing the workout. Each repetition of every set is designed to boost metabolism and build muscle in the least amount of time possible. It'll add several pounds of lean muscle to your frame in just weeks. And that's important not only because you'll look like a stud but also because 1 pound of muscle requires 50 calories per day just to maintain itself on your skeleton, even when it's not engaged in anything physical. Add just 2 pounds of muscle and you'll burn 100 more calories per day even before you exercise.

We've included another element to the chapters in this book: Supershots, which are tricks and techniques for getting more weight-loss bang for your buck. These alternative exercises and technique tips will challenge your muscles in new ways and keep you motivated to work harder at losing your gut for good.

Real Meals are what make the Belly Off! Diet so different from all other diets whose underlying theme is sacrifice and elimination. We took the foods that men cannot live without—steaks, pizza, chili, burgers, and even spaghetti and meatballs—and we developed delicious recipes that'll satisfy your taste buds while sticking to the principles of good nutrition.

Starting with the 7-Day Quick-Start, we give you shopping lists that you can photocopy and take to the grocery store with you. They detail everything you'll need to make the Real Meals in this book. Best of all, each Real Meal will provide you with the right mix of protein (to build muscle and burn calories), fat—yes, tasty fat (to keep you satisfied for a long period of time with fewer cravings!)—and fiber to keep you burning fat and prevent your body from storing it right where you don't want it—your belly.

A KICK IN THE PANTS

Not long after I decided to get back in shape, I went for a long run in my hometown. It was my 47th birthday. I was running past my old high school when I saw the hill that my football team used to run during triple sessions in the August heat. I decided to go for it. Halfway up that weed-choked hill, I was transported back to 1978. I tasted the dust on my teeth and heard the panting of my teammates in my ears. And the voice of our coach, Wild Bill, screaming about how we weren't nearly ready to face North Brunswick in the season opener.

Wild Bill was an old-school football coach, a former linebacker for the Blue Hens of University of Delaware, with a tough-as-nails demeanor, who understood how to motivate teenagers. Rumor has it that he once deposited an insubordinate student into a trash can. (That was long, long ago during a far less litigious era.) Nobody gave Wild Bill grief. And on the practice field, when Billy yelled, people listened.

Full disclosure: Wild Bill is my older cousin Bill Csatari. He's mellowed with age, but you still wouldn't want to go punch-for-punch with him.

Wild Bill's motivational secret involved a little fear, but mostly it was about pride. In 1977, the South River (New Jersey) high school football team lost just one game, 2–0, in the mud against North Brunswick. It was the only blemish on a championship season. And Wild Bill didn't let us forget it the following year during preseason practice. "Remember North Bruns-wick," he'd yell while standing on the back of the blocking sled. "Two to zero," he'd bellow while we were running hills after practice. We watched film of that game countless times. Coach Bill had an annoying habit of clicking a button on the projector to rewind and replay our mistakes for analysis. At the end of this game film, he clicked back and forth, back and forth, over and over again showing the last seconds ticking off the scoreboard, with the score 2–0, just to make sure the memory sunk in. In the locker room before the rematch game, Bill read a telegram that Dallas Cowboys wide receiver Drew Pearson, a South River alumnus, sent to the team: "The man who wins is the man who thinks he can," Pearson wrote. Finally, during warm-ups before that season opener against North Brunswick, Wild Bill placed the game ball from the prior year's loss at midfield.

All those reminders motivated us to work harder; they kept us focused. And I believe they ultimately helped us to avenge that loss with a 14–7 win over the Raiders.

After the game, Wild Bill grabbed a shovel, dug a deep hole, and buried that game ball underneath the stadium goalposts with the entire team (and about half the town) watching.

I walked over that spot during my run on my 47th birthday, wondering if the game ball was still buried there. Or did we dig it up after the season? I had a good laugh as I ran intervals up the stadium stands.

It is my sincere hope that this book will provide you with motivation to revamp your diet, start exer-cising the *right way,* and improve your overall health. And that you'll make those six strategies on page 7 a part of your new lifestyle. It all starts with desire and commitment.

So, what do you say? Are you ready to join the brotherhood of more than 300,000 men who are committed to their health? Are you ready to get into the best shape of your life? And take that belly off?

Then, do this:

Find a photograph of you at your heaviest and tack it someplace where you'll see it often. That's your football buried under the goalposts. It'll serve as a reminder to put down those Twinkies and go for a run. (Many Belly Off! Club members, including Tony Fedora whose "It Works for Me" strategy is mentioned on page 10, say they found the "fat photo" strategy very effective for motivation.)

Next, step on a scale and write your current weight on today's date on a calendar. You'll weigh yourself at the same time of day, and record the result every day. Why? Because a study at the Weight Control and Diabetes Research Center in Providence, Rhode Island, found that people who weighed themselves every day at the same time of day were 82 percent more likely to keep their weight off than people who didn't use a scale. Positive feedback encourages positive action.

Finally, make the following promise on page 14 to yourself. Date it and sign it. Studies show that people who sign a pledge are more likely to follow through with their commitments. It's about accountability.

IT WORKS FOR ME

"Soda and juice are loaded with sugar. I learned to love water; and if I crave juice, I eat a piece of fruit."

—Andrew Lebson, Brooklyn, NY, who lost 100 pounds

THE BELLY OFF! CLUB CODE OF CONDUCT

I PROMISE TO . . .

1. Eat a protein-rich breakfast daily to spark my metabolism and fill me up.

2. Follow the Bodyweight 100 exercise and intervals program and start my day with the Belly Off! 2-Minute Drill.

3. Eat four to six small meals and snacks a day.

4. Replace processed carbohydrates like cakes, cookies, white bread, pasta, and white rice with whole grains, vegetables, and fruits, plus proteins and a little fat.

5. Refrain from drinking alcohol for the next 4 weeks.

Signed _____

Date _____

2

HOW DID WE GET SO FAT?

Knowing What Put the Weight On Can Help You Take It Off

YOU REALLY CAN'T FATHOM how much you can possibly consume in a single day unless you keep track with pencil and paper. Give it a try. I guarantee this little exercise will be an eye-opener.

Last summer our family attended an all-day swimming league championship competition and then grabbed a takeout pizza and a couple of meatball Parmesan sandwiches for dinner on the way home. It was a particularly gluttonous day. As I popped a few Alka-Seltzers that evening, I tried to remember what I had eaten from the time I woke up until *plop-plop fizz-fizz*. I scribbled it all down in a notebook. Here's what I swallowed that Saturday believe it or not:

JEFF'S PRE-BELLY-OFF! ONE-DAY FOOD DIARY

MORNING

One 6-ounce glass of orange juice

Medium Dunkin' Donuts coffee with cream and sugar

One cinnamon raisin bagel with 2 tablespoons cream cheese

Two homemade chocolate chip cookies (to support the swim club bake sale)

One plum

AFTERNOON

Grilled chicken sandwich with cheese on hamburger bun with mayo, lettuce and tomato, pickle, and potato chips

Bowl (1 cup) of pasta salad

One 12-ounce can of grapefruit soda

One 2" square brownie with 1 tablespoon crushed walnuts on top (to support the swim club bake sale)

Hot dog on bun with ketchup and relish that my 2-year-old didn't eat (Confession: I ate it even though I wasn't hungry.)

One 16.9-ounce bottle of Gatorade Tiger Red Drive

Two red Twizzlers

One ice cream sandwich

One bottle of spring water

EVENING

Two slices of cheese pizza

One 12-ounce bottle of Coors Light

Salad with 2 cups greens, $\frac{1}{4}$ cup carrots, $\frac{1}{4}$ cup cherry tomatoes, and croutons; 2 tablespoons french dressing

SNACK

Two dark-chocolate-covered pretzels

One 12-ounce glass of ginger ale

On paper it looks like a heck of a lot of food. And it is—3,795 calories' worth. But, over the course of a day surrounded by a lot of temptation, it's pretty easy to do. If there's a lot of interesting food around, you're going to eat it. And the fund-raising bake sale makes it that much easier to rationalize a few brownies. It adds up, and it often ends up front and center at your belly—our national symbol of overindulgence.

MEET YOUR FAT CELLS

Haven't we all at some point looked in the mirror at our ample abdomens—crafted lovingly over many years of Budweiser and bratwurst—and thought, *Whoo-eee, I look like I swallowed a small child! I ought to do something about that!*

What we're critiquing in that mirror, of course, is how heavy we look. Maybe we have a date coming up. Or we're in the middle of trying on a new suit. Or we realize that beach season is right around the corner and it would be nice to have a Michael Phelps six-pack instead of that Doritos crumb catcher we're currently toting around.

How we look is important to our self-esteem, to our careers, to our love lives. But, there is a more important reason to be concerned with shedding that gut. It's simply not healthy. Let's take a peek at your potbelly to see why.

The average man—that's you—is home to about 30 billion fat cells. If you thought of them as extremely tiny water balloons, you wouldn't be far off. But instead of being filled with water, they are filled with oily fats, technically called lipids. Our bodies produce these fats, and we also get them from food.

Your fat cells are designed to be a reservoir for energy when you need it. Problem is, you get more fat than you need for energy, and those cells expand like balloons and can divide, creating even more repositories for lipids. These extra cells don't go anywhere. You can shrink them but you can't get rid of them, which is why losing weight can be so tough once you've ballooned up. And unfortunately, unwanted fat tends to collect in your abdomen and lower chest region—between the nipples and the navel—creating an apple-shaped body. Sometimes this fat congregates about the hips, butt, and thighs, creating a pear shape. Most men, however, fall into the apple-shape category of fat storage, which is the most dangerous.

Give your gut a little poke right now. Does it jiggle? Is it soft like pudding or could you bounce a baseball off of it? (I'm assuming you're *not* the owner of a rock-hard six-pack like the one you had when you were, say, 10—remember?) Soft and protruding or hard and protruding. Those are the two basic types of male potbellies, and one is much worse to have than the other. The soft kind is mostly made up of *subcutaneous* fat, meaning it's located just under the skin in front of the abdominal muscles. Nobody likes this fat.

FAT FACT

197

The number of times you'd have to run the length of a football field to burn off the 1,460 calories in a 10-piece order of McDonald's Fried Chicken Selects Premium Breast Strips with Spicy Buffalo Sauce

You want it to vanish. Still, it's not as bad to have as the other kind.

The round and hard type of belly is made up of *visceral* fat, which resides behind the abs and forms around the *viscera,* another name for your internal organs. Fat that's hard up against your most crucial body parts like this is not a good thing. Visceral fat secretes harmful juices—compounds that raise blood pressure, hormones that lead to high blood sugar, and a particularly dangerous chemical called interleukin-6 that's associated with inflamed arteries. All you have to know is that the bigger and harder your belly, the larger your visceral fat cells and the more active they are at secreting these harmful juices.

A protruding belly of 40 inches or more is one of the markers of a condition known as *metabolic syndrome* or *prediabetes.* The other telltale signs are high blood pressure, high triglycerides (fat in your blood), high blood sugar, and low HDL (good) cholesterol. Having a big belly and any two other markers means you have metabolic syndrome and should see your doctor for a blood test.

According to the Centers for Disease Control and Prevention, 54 million Americans are living with prediabetes, and the incidence is growing faster among men than among women. Prediabetes or metabolic syndrome is associated with every major age-related illness, including erectile dysfunction, Alzheimer's disease, blindness, kidney failure, cancer, and heart disease. Untreated, prediabetes will turn into full-blown type 2 diabetes, also known as adult-onset diabetes. In fact, having this condition increases your chances of developing diabetes fivefold, and it doubles your risk of a heart attack.

What exactly is diabetes? Basically, it's your body's inability to process sugar properly. But to fully understand this disease, it helps to know how the body uses food for energy.

A quick biology lesson: When your body digests food, it turns the carbohydrates—that is, the sugars and starches—into *glucose,* the official term for blood sugar. Glucose is the fuel that powers your cells. But

FAT FACT
A protruding belly of 40 inches or more is one of the markers of prediabetes.

Get a sneak peek of our
Spring Fashion &
see everything that's new this season

Friday & Saturday, February 20 & 21

Doors open at 10 a.m.
*First 300 shoppers will
receive a scratch-off card
for 20%, 30% or 40%
OFF entire purchase!

Stein Mart®
Once you go you get it.

Stein Mart Mailing Center
804 Greenbrier Circle, Suite C
Chesapeake, VA 23320

1-888-STEIN MART • www.steinmart.com

PRESORTED
FIRST CLASS MAIL
US POSTAGE
PAID
STEIN MART

Requested In-Home 2/17/09

Virginia Riegel
48 Creek Rdg
Pittsford NY 14534-4404

get up
& go!

See new spring fashions that have just arrived.

Once you **go** you get it.

This Friday & Saturday, be one of the first lucky shoppers to receive a

Scratch & Save card.*

Save at least **20%** or even **30%** or **40% OFF** your entire purchase.

*While supplies last.

Stein Mart ®

here's the key thing to know about glucose: It can't get into your body's cells on its own. It needs help from *insulin,* a hormone that is secreted by your pancreas. Acting like a key to a lock, insulin opens the door to certain cells and moves sugar from the blood into organs like the brain, liver, and muscles. It is also insulin's job to deal with the fats we get from foods like meat, dairy products, and vegetable oils. Insulin transports these *fatty acids* from the blood-stream into the body's tissues, where they are either used for energy or stored for future use.

The pancreas is an unsung hero of all this, and it deserves our praise. But the way we Americans eat often confuses this highly efficient organ. Here's how: Let's say you have a typical American lunch of a cheeseburger and large french fries and a 20-ounce cola, and then maybe you partake in a slice of choco-late cake because it's Linda's 30th birthday in the office next door and you want to be a "team player." Suddenly, your system has much more energy than it can use right away, so insulin moves in to help. It hauls that surplus glucose into your liver, where it's turned into *glycogen,* and it takes the fatty acids from the blood to your fat cells, where they're saved as *triglycerides* (blood fats).

This flood of insulin drives your blood sugar lower, which makes you feel hungry again. For what? For still more starches. A package of cookies, perhaps, or a candy bar. The cravings are similar to those a drug addict or alcoholic experiences. And the process continues. Blood sugar jacks up from the new carbs, the pancreas dutifully responds with more insulin, and so on. Over time, this recurrence can lead to insulin resistance. You need more and more insulin to do the same job.

"The high-blood-glucose response to a high-carb diet is almost a normal response to an abnormal situation," explains Ron Raab, past vice president of the International Diabetes Federation. "We've largely created this illness (diabetes)" by the way we now eat. Eventually, the insulin manufactured by the pancreas becomes ineffective—that's diabetes. Once

FAT FACT
It's Your Girth Day: People consume an average of 236 more calories on Saturday than on any given weekday, according to a study in the journal *Obesity.*

you have diabetes, you must now closely monitor your blood sugar levels and manage blood sugar with oral insulin or injections. If blood sugar isn't managed effectively, you can lose 5 to 10 years of your life span and put yourself at great risk for blindness, nerve damage, amputation, impotence, kidney disease, stroke, and heart disease. Now you know why you should appreciate your pancreas.

Belly fat is also a major risk factor for cancer. A study in the *New England Journal of Medicine* concluded that virtually all forms of cancer are more prevalent in people with fatty bodies, and 15 percent of all cancer deaths could be tied to being overweight. What's fat got to do with cancer? Easy answer: Fat upsets the body's natural hormonal balance, making tissue an easier host for tumors.

As if that weren't enough, an unchecked fat belly automatically builds an even fatter belly by changing the very core of what makes you a man—testosterone. That's the male hormone tied to red blood cell

MEASURE YOUR RISK
Two Easy Self-Tests That Will Help You Take Charge

THE TAPE TEST

Take off your shirt and lower your pants so your middle hangs out. Wrap a soft measuring tape around your abdomen so that the bottom of the tape touches the tops of your hipbones. Standing in front of a mirror will help you make sure the tape is positioned correctly, parallel with the floor. Don't suck in your gut. Let it all hang out. Stand straight and exhale as you pull the tape taut against the skin (without compressing the skin). Look at the number corresponding with the "0" on the tape—that's your waist measurement. A waist size of 40 inches or over for men and 35 inches or over for women is considered high risk for every ugly disease we mentioned above.

BMI, OR BODY MASS INDEX

The BMI is a formula for measuring your body fat based on your height and weight. There's a mathematical formula for figuring BMI, but the easiest way is to use a free online calculator. Plug "body mass index" into your search engine or type this National Institutes of Health Web address into your browser: www.nhlbisupport.com/bmi/. Enter your height and weight, and the calculator will figure out your BMI in seconds. A BMI of 30 or greater indicates obesity, 25 to 29.9 means overweight, and 18.5 to 24.9 is normal weight.

production, muscle development, and sexual functioning. A 20-year study tracking 584 men published recently in the *Journal of Clinical Endocrinology and Metabolism* found that a 4-point increase in body mass index—a calculation used to determine obesity—accelerates your natural decline in testosterone by 10 years. This shortcut dip in the male hormone corresponded to an average gain of 30 pounds for a man of average height.

Know what 30 pounds feels like? Grab two 15-pound dumbbells or two bowling balls and walk around for 10 minutes. Pretty tough. Well, that's the extra work that you're asking your heart to do 24/7 when you are 30 pounds over your ideal weight.

See Measure Your Risk (opposite) for two simple early-warning home tests to gauge your girth. Use them as an incentive to act now.

WHAT THE HECK HAPPENED?

I could fill this entire chapter on the dangers of visceral fat and obesity, but I think you get the bleak picture already. Instead, let's learn how we as a nation got so fat. That knowledge will help you set your sights on how to get rid of your gut and live a healthier and longer life.

WE EAT TOO MUCH FOOD

A history lesson: In 1960 the average American man weighed 166 pounds. The average woman weighed 140. Today, the average man weighs 191 pounds, and the average woman checks in at nearly what that dude wearing the skinny tie and horn-rimmed glasses used to weigh—164. Amazing, no? But those are just averages. The scariest statistics can be found at the top of the scale: The number of Americans who are considered obese—essentially 30 or more pounds overweight—has almost doubled to around 40 million. All this corresponds nicely with the increase in the

American food consumption since the Summer of Love. Back in the 1970s, the average man swallowed about 2,450 calories a day, according to the National Health and Nutrition Examination Surveys. Now that figure is over 2,700—an increase of nearly 10 percent!

Are you part of that national trend? A simple at-home exercise will paint a clear picture of both how much you eat and exactly what you're putting in your mouth. Keep a food diary for 3 days. Diary? Okay, now before you say, "I don't do diaries," consider this: Keeping a food diary is one of the most effective ways to lose your gut. The simple act of writing down what you eat each day can double the amount of weight you lose, according to one of the largest and longest-running weight-loss maintenance studies ever conducted. When doctors at the Kaiser Permanente Center for Health Research in Portland, Oregon, compared the different approaches to maintaining weight loss of 1,685 overweight or obese adults over 20 months, they found that people who kept track of their meals lost twice as much weight as those who didn't.

Try keeping a food diary for even just one day as I did (page 16). It will be as surprising for you as it was for me. Your diary doesn't have to be a formal chart. Scribble it on a napkin. Write it on a calendar. Or, if you believe it will help you to use a food diary as an official tool for your weight-loss effort, make photocopies of the 7-day sample diary starting on page 30 to work with. It's the process of reflecting on what we eat that helps us to become aware of our habits and hopefully change our behaviors, says Keith Bachman, MD, a researcher at Kaiser Permanente's Weight Management Initiative.

OUR PORTIONS ARE ENORMOUS

Have you gone to an Italian restaurant lately? (Hey, I'm not picking on Italians—someone in my kitchen would throw a cannoli at me.) Just think about what you see on your plate after you've noshed on that basket of garlic bread and the antipasto, and

FIT FACT

In a study of 1685 overweight people, those who kept a food diary lost twice as much weight as those who didn't track their intake.

your server finally brings the spaghetti. A mound of pasta—easily three or more servings on that plate—with meatballs the size of oranges on top. There could be a Mount Vesuvius of 2,400 calories sitting there—and that's before you get to the tiramisu. If you're like me, you'll eat it all. Thanks to Mom and Dad, who grew up during the post-Great Depression years and taught us to clean our plates. Sop up gravy with another slice of Wonder Bread. There are children starving in Africa, you know.

Mom and Dad shouldn't feel guilty for laying guilt on us. Blame the savvy marketers who created the enormous portions and the extra-value meals. The U.S. Department of Agriculture has documented this unhealthy growth in food portion size:

- In 1957, a serving of popcorn at the drive-in was 3 cups. Today a medium-size popcorn at the multiplex is 16 cups.

- In 1957, 1 ounce of cooked ground beef made up your typical hamburger. Today the average hamburger is 6 ounces.

- Muffins were tiny in 1957, about 1½ ounces. Now they typically weigh in at 8 ounces and pack 400 calories.

- A large soda in 1957 measured 8 fluid ounces compared with 32 ounces in 1997, or often 64 ounces today.

Thanks to the big plates we're getting when we eat out, we've become a culture of "more is better" where "supersize me" is our mantra when we order. And this has confused our sense of a proper serving size. Studies show that when people are asked to describe how much they eat, they invariably underestimate. Big time. Then there is the buffet phenomenon. When we are faced with an abundance of food and food choices, we tend to serve ourselves

IT WORKS FOR ME

"On average, a restaurant will give you double, if not triple, the amount of food you really need to feel satisfied. Try this: When the server brings the food, ask for a to-go box, and put half of your meal in it before you begin eating. You'll eat the right amount and have a ready-made lunch for tomorrow."

—Kirk Ward, Charlotte, NC, who lost 70 pounds

more than we need. One Rutgers University study measured the amount of food people served themselves from a breakfast buffet. Then they compared the results to a similar study conducted 19 years earlier. The recent study participants served themselves 16 percent more toast with jelly, 43 percent more orange juice, 28 percent more milk for their cereal, and 19 percent more cornflakes than the similar group did nearly two decades earlier.

Even diet experts who should know better screw up portion sizes. In a recent Cornell University study, nutritionists who were asked to serve themselves ice cream at a party using large bowls and spoons dished out about 31 percent more than those who were given smaller bowls and spoons. Cookies 'n' Cream and Moosetracks have a miraculous way of tricking us into seeing our bowls as half empty.

SIZE MATTERS
You Don't Have to Count Calories If You Can Spot a Real Portion When You See One

I don't care if you're a hungry cowboy, the Big Texan is not a meal meant for a human. At 72 ounces (that's 4½ pounds), this specially cut top sirloin, grilled at the Big Texan Steak Ranch on old Route 66 in Amarillo, epitomizes (elephantizes?) all that is wrong with the way we view restaurant food and good value. The meal, by the way, is free if you can eat it all—including the baked potato, salad, dinner roll, and shrimp cocktail—in less than an hour. A Bengal tiger did it in 90 seconds. No less than 40,000 people have attempted the big beef meal, and some 7,000 gluttonous souls have succeeded.

You don't need to order in Amarillo to eat too much. Most restaurant meals, and even those we cook for ourselves at home, are abnormal in size, by nutritional standards.

To keep calories, carbs, and fat in check, it helps to be able to eyeball a serving of food and gauge how much it exceeds the normal portion size. You can save that extra part for the doggy bag. Here are some guidelines for normal serving sizes.

3 to 4 ounces of meat (the recommended healthy size for a meal) = a deck of playing cards or a bar of soap

8 ounces of meat = a thin paperback book

3 ounces of fish = a checkbook

1 ounce of cheese = 4 dice

A medium potato = a computer mouse

2 tablespoons of peanut butter = a ping-pong ball

An average bagel = a hockey puck

ADDED SUGARS LURK EVERYWHERE

Not only are we Americans eating more food, but we are eating more starchy carbohydrates such as processed grains, potatoes, corn, and sugar. Unlike protein, fat, and fiber—which have little if any impact on blood sugar—these starches quickly break down in our bodies and cause a fast increase in our blood-sugar levels, which in turn causes an insulin spike.

Scientists have devised a system, called the Glycemic Load, or GL, that rates foods based on how they affect blood sugar and insulin level. Pancakes, for example, have a high glycemic load of 39; orange soda, 23; a baked russet potato, 26. Watermelon, even though it is sweet, has a very low glycemic load of 4 because of its high water volume. Generally, it's wiser to choose lower-GL carbohydrates, the ones that produce smaller fluctuations in blood sugar and insulin levels. High GL foods have a rating of 20 or more; low GL foods a rating of 10 or less. For a chart of Glycemic Load values for select foods, see "Understanding Glycemic Load" in the appendix on page 323.

Today the average American consumes about 154 pounds of added sugars per year, about 45 pounds more than he ate in the 1950s. Why? We're not just adding more table sugar to our coffee. From 1970 to 1997, the availability of corn sweeteners increased about 350 percent. Food manufacturers started adding sugar to foods in the form of high-fructose corn syrup (HFCS) because it's cheap to produce and makes for highly profitable products. It's everywhere, not just in candy, cookies, and cakes. HFCS is in soda, juices, breads, condiments, frozen dinners, and cereals. During that same period of time, our consumption of grains and cereal products jumped from about 136 pounds per person to more than 198 pounds, according to the USDA. That's problematic because most of those grains come in the form of highly refined flours found in white bread, pastas, and breakfast cereals, and they act just like the sweeteners do, causing blood sugar to spike fast.

FAT FACT

The 27 grams of sugar in an 8.3-ounce can of Red Bull may be enough to temporarily inhibit your body's ability to burn fat.

FAT FACT

5.8

Number of beers the average man drinks in a week

8

Number of alcoholic drinks the average man has each week

60

Number of gallons of alcohol the average man drinks in a year

Watch out for hidden sources found in everything from juices to cereal bars. Spot them by reading food labels and knowing the names of the sweet stuff:

- High-fructose corn syrup
- Glucose
- Sucrose
- Maltose
- Dextrose
- Honey
- Fruit concentrate
- Natural cane sugar

These foods are typically loaded with hidden sugars:

- Yogurt
- Jelly
- Canned fruit
- Spaghetti sauce
- Soups
- Sausage
- Salad dressings
- Peanut butter
- Crackers
- Frozen desserts

WE DRINK OUR CALORIES

Soft drinks are the leading source of calories in the average American's diet, accounting for nearly 1 in every 10 calories consumed, according to a 2005 study. We drink 52 gallons per person per year. The average American consumes almost 60 pounds of high-fructose corn syrup per year, according to the

U.S. Department of Agriculture. And much of it comes from soda. A 12-ounce can of soda contains 13 teaspoons of high-fructose corn syrup. Soft drinks are so stealthy in this caloric war because the brain interprets liquids as less filling than solid foods. Case in point: When Purdue University researchers, in a 2007 study, gave subjects foods in both liquid and solid forms, the people consumed many more calories on the days when they ate food in liquid form than when they ate solid food.

Fruit juice is no better than soda and it may even be worse; it sounds natural and healthful, so we may rationalize drinking more of it. How much more healthful can you get than drinking vitamin C–rich orange juice or the new favorite, pomegranate juice? Well, unless your OJ has a lot of pulp, it's like injecting pure sugar directly into your veins. Liquid doesn't have to be broken down as whole fruit does, so the sugar—even though it's the same type—goes directly into the bloodstream. That's why eating whole fruit is a much smarter option. There's fiber in the skin of an apple and in the white fleshy part of an orange, which slows down the sugar infusion because it takes longer for your intestines to process it. A 2007 study in the *International Journal of Obesity* reported that people who substituted a piece of whole fruit for fruit juice with their lunch reduced their daily calories by as much as 20 percent. Likewise, when participants ate cheese instead of drinking milk, they saw a similar reduction in calories consumed. Solids take longer to process. What's more, the researchers found that the act of chewing stimulates satiety hormones better than swallowing liquid does. If you can't stop drinking juice cold turkey, do what I do: Buy OJ with pulp and cut it with water. You'll effectively halve your calories and dramatically reduce the blood-sugar rush.

Here's a case against beer: There is a reason we call big guts "beer bellies" after all. Beer is loaded with carbohydrates, which, as we've learned, create fat. You don't get off the hook so easily switching to light or low-carb beers; they still have alcohol in them.

FAT FACT

17

Number of teaspoons of sugar in a typical 20-ounce soda

FAT FACT

73

Percent increase in
calories consumed
when you supersize
a fast-food meal of
medium fries and
medium cola to a
large of both,
according to a
University of
Wisconsin study

And alcohol impairs your body from burning fat. In one study, Swiss researchers gave eight healthy men the equivalent in alcohol of about five regular beers. They determined that the alcohol slowed the subjects' ability to burn fat by 36 percent.

Here's the chemical process that leads to a beer belly: You take a swig of beer. Within seconds, your stomach starts absorbing about 20 percent of the alcohol and sends it directly into your bloodstream. The rest is absorbed in your intestines. The alcohol in your blood is broken down in your liver, where it creates waste products called *acetate* and *acetaldehyde*. Acetate and acetaldehyde signal your body to stop burning fat. At the same time, your body starts making fat from another waste product of alcohol, called *acetyl CoA*. Double whammy. More fat is made that can't be burned.

The same thing happens when you drink wine and hard liquors such as vodka, gin, and whiskey that don't even contain carbohydrates. And when you mix hard liquor with non-diet soda, juice, and other high-fructose mixers, you essentially turn a no-carb drink into a high-carb drink that'll lead to fat storage in your belly.

Now, you might be thinking, "What about all you've read about the health benefits of booze?" True, beer and wine have been shown to contain substances called flavonoids that may ward off coronary artery disease, hypertension, and even dementia. A substance called resveratrol, found in the skins of grapes used to make red wine, has been shown to protect the linings of arteries. But doctors say you lose the health benefits of drinking alcohol once you down three or more drinks. You have to ask yourself, how easy is it to limit yourself to just a drink or two at parties or restaurant dinners? That's the point where the scale tips in the other direction. A large study of middle-age people several years ago found that men who had more than three drinks a day were 50 percent more likely to develop diabetes than men who had just one drink per week. The same study showed that men who downed 14 hard liquor drinks in a week were 80 percent more likely to develop diabetes than men who drank beer or wine but no hard liquor. Of course, we also need to consider our favorite drinking buddy: food. (See "Bar Chart" below.) Alcohol and eating go hand in hand.

WE DON'T EXERCISE, OUR METABOLISM SLOWS, OUR MUSCLES SHRINK

We have much to look forward to as we get older—ear hair, bifocals, a prescription for Cialis. Add a slower metabolism to your list. It's a fact of life—the older you get, the fewer calories you burn. A 180-pound man in his forties burns on average about 12 fewer calories per hour at rest than a man of the same weight in his twenties. That means he ends the day with 288 more calories than the younger guy—unless he does something about it. Researchers have estimated that the decline continues at the rate of 2 to 4 percent per decade after age 40. Conspiring to make

(continued on page 35)

BAR CHART
Last Call for Pub Grub

Cutting out alcohol is one of the most effective ways to lose your gut. Why? Because alcohol is high in calories, containing about 7 calories per gram, which isn't far from the 9 calories in a gram of fat. But there's another reason to eliminate booze for a month. With beer comes pub grub. It's a fact that when you drink, you want to snack on fatty, salty stuff—from buffalo wings to Goldfish crackers. And how many times, after leaving the bar, have you made a pit stop at White Castle for 10 Original Sliders? Admit it. We've got the videotapes.

Just how bad is bar food? Have a look.

TWO BEERS WITH . . .	CALORIES	FAT (G)
1 cup peanuts	1,146	72
7 buffalo wings	1,028	44
8 nachos supreme	861	31
4 fried cheese sticks	512	12
30 corn chips	447	9
10 mini-hamburgers	1,350	70

BLOAT CHECK: YOUR 7-DAY FOOD DIARY
Fill It Out to Focus on What You're Eating and How Much

Keeping a food diary is a useful exercise to help you become hyper-aware of what you put in your mouth. And it can identify binge triggers, like alcohol or foods, or certain types of restaurants and even friends with whom you tend to eat and drink more. As mentioned earlier, clinical studies show that people who make the effort to write down what they eat every day lose more weight than those who don't keep track. The practice is very simple. Make photo copies of pages 30 through 33 and keep them in a notebook or on a clipboard. Record everything you eat and when you eat it. Do it after every meal or at the end of the day. Doesn't matter. Try it for at least 3 days, and you'll recognize its power to change habits. It will be an enlightening exercise.

DAY 1

Before noon   **Afternoon**   **After 5 p.m.**

_____   _____   _____

_____   _____   _____

_____   _____   _____

_____   _____   _____

_____   _____   _____

_____   _____   _____

_____   _____   _____

DAY 2

Before noon   **Afternoon**   **After 5 p.m.**

_____   _____   _____

_____   _____   _____

_____   _____   _____

_____   _____   _____

_____   _____   _____

_____   _____   _____

_____   _____   _____

DAY 3

Before noon   **Afternoon**   **After 5 p.m.**

_____   _____   _____

_____   _____   _____

_____   _____   _____

_____   _____   _____

_____   _____   _____

_____   _____   _____

_____   _____   _____

DAY 4

Before noon   **Afternoon**   **After 5 p.m.**

_____   _____   _____

_____   _____   _____

_____   _____   _____

_____   _____   _____

_____   _____   _____

_____   _____   _____

_____   _____   _____

DAY 5

Before noon   **Afternoon**   **After 5 p.m.**

_____   _____   _____

_____   _____   _____

_____   _____   _____

_____   _____   _____

_____   _____   _____

_____   _____   _____

DAY 6

Before noon   **Afternoon**   **After 5 p.m.**

_____   _____   _____

_____   _____   _____

_____   _____   _____

_____   _____   _____

_____   _____   _____

_____   _____   _____

_____   _____   _____

DAY 7

Before noon   **Afternoon**   **After 5 p.m.**

_____   _____   _____

_____   _____   _____

_____   _____   _____

_____   _____   _____

_____   _____   _____

_____   _____   _____

REAL GUYS—REAL RESULTS

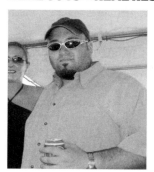

BEFORE:
340
POUNDS

AFTER:
185
POUNDS

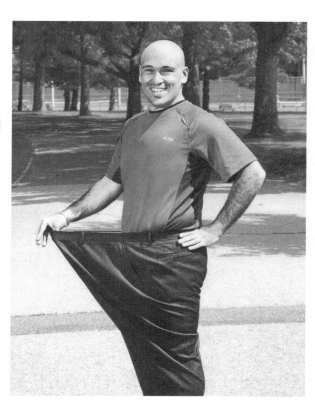

"I wanted to stop avoiding mirrors."

VITALS: Brian Spar, 30, Long Beach, NY

OCCUPATION: Veterinarian

HEIGHT: 5'9"

LESSON LEARNED: Self-honesty. Before, I'd convince myself I wasn't that big or unhealthy.

Spar, who's a self-proclaimed cheeseburger addict and couch potato, saw his extra weight from childhood barrel out of control when he moved to London for veterinary school. He skipped breakfast, and his diet consisted mostly of beer, fried foods, and a liter of Coke a day. When the scale topped 340 pounds, he had trouble breathing.

THE TURNING POINT

The newly engaged Spar saw a framed photo of his large self on his dad's desk. "It was embarrassing. I decided to grow up and get my life under control." He started walking for 30 minutes three times a week. He ditched fried fare and sugary treats and switched to whole-grain bread.

LIFE IN THE FIT LANE

Spar now begins his day with a hearty bowl of oatmeal along with egg whites. He eats healthy snacks during the day and high-protein foods with vegetables at lunch and dinner. Spar hits the gym 5 days a week for 45 minutes of cardio and weight lifting. When it's warm, he runs 5 miles at the beach once a week.

THE REWARD

After trimming his physique, Spar decided to put his newly defined body to the test by running a 5-K. He finished with a time of 28:51. His running continues to improve, and he will run a half marathon this year. Now when he shops for clothes, he actually enjoys it. His waistline was 50 inches; today, he wears a trim 32.

SPAR'S BEST BELLY OFF! TIPS

● Ease into the new you. Motivation is great, but changing your diet too quickly will increase cravings and set you up for failure.

● Try changing one food group at a time.

● Look beyond the menu. If you're going to eat in a restaurant, ask the server how the meals are prepared. If the menu says a dish is sautéed, it probably means it's smothered in butter. Ask the chef to use olive oil instead.

● Find a workout buddy. Working out with my wife helped me stay motivated to keep up my program. And it improved our relationship and made us both feel better.

burning extra calories even more difficult is the fact that most of us have jobs that don't require physical exertion, especially as we advance our careers. According to researchers at the University of North Carolina at Wilmington, people who start a typical sedentary office job will gain an average of 16 pounds in the first 8 months.

And while you are burning less energy sitting at that desk, your muscles are shrinking. Between the ages of 30 and 50, the average man loses 6 pounds of muscle. No wonder you and your classmates at your 15th high school reunion looked so different from your graduation pictures. Remember that muscle burns 50 more calories per day than fat does. So when you have less of it, your metabolism slows even more. If you don't scale back your calorie consumption or increase your activity level as you get older, you *will* gain weight. Guaranteed. And we do. In our 30s and 40s, career and family obligations have a way of making it more difficult for us to find time to take care of our bodies. And I don't know about you, but my taste for fine dining and good wine has grown over the years, and the opportunities to enjoy both—on the job and socially—have increased exponentially.

So now, after reading all this, you may be thinking, "I'm doomed." Human biology and American food culture have saddled me with a life-threatening potbelly that's going to be extremely difficult to get rid of.

Don't worry. Understanding how our nation got so fat is a crucial tool to help you sidestep the land mines in your own life. In the next chapter, you'll learn the five pillars of the Belly Off! Diet and how to immediately start making them a part of your healthier lifestyle.

SUPERSHOT
Use Small Plates

Reduce the amount of food you eat by using smaller plates. Studies show that people are programmed to eat more when they use large plates or dishes that have patterns on them.

3

HOW THE BELLY OFF! DIET WORKS

The New Scientific Evidence Behind Your Code of Conduct

Why am I so soft in the middle,
when the rest of my life is so hard?
—Paul Simon

WELL, **IF YOU READ** the last chapter and tried keeping a food diary, you should have a pretty good answer to Mr. Simon's lament.

We men eat a lot of food. We eat a lot of the wrong kinds of foods— starchy carbs and lots of sugars that go right to our guts. We eat them at the wrong times of the day— rarely early and mostly late. Meat loaf and mashed potatoes with gravy and dinner rolls, followed by a side of chocolate frosted cake a la mode, for dinner at 8 p.m. This major infiltration of calories sits there in your belly, while your pancreas works overtime, and your thumb works the TV remote. Then you go to sleep, while your digestive system pulls a night shift.

Food in—less energy out.
Fat happens.

While it may seem that the Pringles are stacked against you, there's a way out of this mess.

You didn't forget your promise, did you?

You've already crossed a huge hurdle even before picking up a fork and lacing your running shoes: You've signed the Belly Off! Club Code of Conduct, a commitment to yourself to follow the principles of the Belly Off! Diet—and to stick with them. Here they are again—five simple rules. Easy to follow. Proven by real guys. Backed by science.

THE BELLY OFF! CLUB CODE OF CONDUCT

I PROMISE TO . . .

1. Eat a protein-rich breakfast daily to spark my metabolism and fill me up.

2. Follow the Bodyweight 100 exercise and intervals program and start my day with the Belly Off! 2-Minute Drill.

3. Eat four to six small meals and snacks a day.

4. Replace processed carbohydrates like cakes, cookies, white bread, pasta, and rice with whole grains, vegetables, and fruits, plus proteins and a little fat.

5. Refrain from drinking alcohol for the next 4 weeks.

There you have it. Eat often (and well!), starting with breakfast, cut out empty carbs, and exercise scientifically. Those are the basic principles of the Belly Off! Diet. Each one is designed to amp up your metabolism, which is your body's fat-burning furnace. Each one has been proven successful by the men who've graced our Belly Off! Club page in *Men's*

Health over the past 8 years. Each one is easy to incorporate into your lifestyle for the rest of your life. Follow them religiously for the next 4 weeks, and you will start to see results—less weight, more energy, fewer cravings—within 5 days.

Later in this book, you'll learn simple tricks to stick to these rules, plus hundreds of ways to make eating and exercising even more effective at getting rid of belly fat. Here's the science behind the five rules that will help you lose up to 20 pounds in 30 days.

RULE #1: EAT BREAKFAST

Eating breakfast is like putting kindling on the fire of your metabolism. Like Grandma said, it's the most important meal of the day—*now eat your mush!* Resolve never to skip the morning meal again. University of Massachusetts Medical School researchers found that men who skip breakfast are 4½ times more likely to be obese than those who eat it. Try to eat something within 90 minutes of waking up.

"Not eating breakfast may reduce your metabolic rate by up to 10 percent," according to Leslie Bonci, a registered dietitian and director of sports nutrition at the University of Pittsburgh Medical Center.

Dieters often think they are doing themselves a favor by skipping breakfast. But that strategy can actually sabotage weight-loss efforts. When you don't eat breakfast, you are effectively fasting for 15 to 20 hours, considering you haven't eaten since dinner and you spent the night sleeping. If you don't *break that fast,* your body won't produce the enzymes needed to metabolize fat to lose weight. Your body slips into starvation mode, hoarding fat in fear of a famine that never comes. Later in the day when you are ravenous, you'll simply open the fridge and stuff your face. Studies show that breakfast skippers tend to replace calories during the day with mindless snacking and they're often so hungry that they'll binge at lunch and dinner.

In a 2008 study, researchers at Virginia Commonwealth University found that dieters who regularly

IT WORKS FOR ME

"Always keep something in your stomach so your body doesn't go into starvation mode and store fat."

—Darren Geffre, Los Lunas, NM, who lost 92 pounds

ate a protein-rich, 600-calorie breakfast lost significantly more weight in 8 months than those who consumed only 300 calories and a quarter of the protein. Turns out, the big breakfast eaters, who lost 40 pounds, had an easier time sticking with the diet even though both groups were prescribed about the same number of total daily calories.

Protein at breakfast is clearly important. Another study published in 2008 in the *British Journal of Nutrition* found that eating extra protein for breakfast leads to feelings of fullness that can last throughout the day. The study, conducted by researchers at the University of Kansas Medical Center and Purdue University, scored the feelings of fullness of nine men who were given normal amounts of protein and extra protein at breakfast, lunch, and dinner or spaced evenly throughout the day. The men were tested while on a regular diet and then while eating a calorie-restricted diet. The results showed that the men on the calorie-restricted diet had their hunger satisfied longest when they ate extra protein at breakfast. "Our findings suggest that people trying to lose weight should eat more protein for breakfast to help them avoid overeating the rest of the day," says study author Heather Leidy, MD, of the University of Kansas Medical Center.

Here's an example of a good high-protein breakfast: Have two scrambled eggs, one or two slices of Canadian bacon, and an 8-ounce glass of low-fat milk. Top that off with a mid-morning snack of a cup of yogurt or whole-wheat toast with peanut butter.

So eat your eggs, turkey bacon, and whole-wheat toast when you have the time. (See Real Meals recipes in Chapter 7.) Don't be afraid of a little saturated fat, either. If you're healthy, there's no scientific reason that natural foods containing some saturated fat can't be part of your diet. Full disclosure: The kind of breakfast in the study does take time to prepare—time you may not have in the morning. So when you're rushed, slather some peanut butter on a banana, eat a protein bar, or roll a slice of deli turkey

FIT FACT

23

Percentage reduction in heart attack risk if you eat two to four servings of fish per week, according to an analysis of the eating habits of more than 220,000 people for 11 years by scientists at Northwestern University

in a slice of Swiss cheese. Leave a bowl of fruit or bags of trail mix near your front door so you can grab them as you leave. Cold pizza can be breakfast, friend. Don't skip this meal. *Capisce?*

RULE #2: EXERCISE INTELLIGENTLY

Study after study has shown that dieting alone rarely works, and weight loss is impossible to sustain without some exercise. That's why we're making it part of your daily morning routine, like shaving and letting the dog out. The Belly Off! 2-Minute Drill, a circuit of strength and cardio calisthenics detailed in Chapter 4, is designed to start your day off on the right foot. It sparks your fat-burners after a night of sleep and serves as an alarm bell to remind you that the key to weight loss is keeping your metabolism revving high all day long. Plus, studies have shown that athletes who work out first thing in the morning stoke their metabolisms higher and longer and burn more calories throughout the day than exercisers who did their workouts at the end of the day.

Ideally, use the 2-Minute Drill as a warmup to a full morning workout—and you'll be done for the day. But if you can't find time for a full workout in the morning, that's okay. Just do the drill when you wake up, and do your longer workout in the afternoon or evening. What's critical is that you fit in three or four Bodyweight routines per week and two or three workouts of high-intensity interval training. As mentioned earlier, the combination of muscle-building moves and cardio-enhancing intervals has a powerful effect on belly fat. Skeletal muscle burns more calories than fat does, so it behooves you to add muscle mass. When it comes to cardio training, new research shows that intervals— short bursts of intense exertion interspersed with periods of slower activity—burn fat and improve fitness more quickly than long, moderate bouts of exercise. And intervals trigger an afterburn effect similar to weight lifting, keeping your body churning through calories long after you've hit the showers.

In a study by a researcher in the Department of Human Health and Nutritional Sciences at the University of Guelph in Canada, exercisers were asked to ride a stationary bike every other day for 2 weeks. They alternated between 10 sets of 4-minute bursts of riding at 90 percent effort with 2-minute slow-pedaling rest intervals. Researcher Jason Talanian found that the subjects experienced an increase in fat used during the intervals as well as an increase in a muscle enzyme that burns fat. What's more, after interval training, the amount of fat the subjects burned in an hour of even moderate pedaling also increased—by 36 percent! So intense intervals had the effect of turbocharging even easy-level exercise.

RULE #3: EAT FOUR TO SIX TIMES A DAY

Eat three regular meals and one or two smart snacks every day to keep your metabolism stoked. A study in the *American Journal of Epidemiology* found that men who ate this frequently were half as likely to become overweight compared with men who ate just three or fewer times daily. Spacing your calories throughout the day by eating something every 3 hours or so keeps blood sugar levels even and controls the release of insulin that can cause your body to store more calories as fat. When you eat less frequently or skip meals, your metabolic furnace goes cold, triggering your body's primal instinct to slow down, conserve energy, and store fat. By contrast, every time you eat, your metabolism speeds up to digest the food.

Your eating schedule might look like this:

6:30 A.M.	**BREAKFAST**
10:00 A.M.	**SNACK**
1:00 P.M.	**LUNCH**
4:00 P.M.	**SNACK**
6:30 P.M.	**DINNER**
8:30 P.M.	**SNACK (OPTIONAL)**

Whenever possible, prepare your own meals to reduce your need to visit fast-food spots. That way you have better control over ingredients, since fast food tends to be high in calories, carbohydrates, sodium, and fat. US Department of Agriculture scientists studying American eating habits found that men eat on average 500 more calories on days when they consume fast foods compared with days when they make their own meals. "Cooking creates a personal connection to food and gives you an intimate understanding of what you're ultimately consuming," says Bob Harper, a personal trainer and star of the TV reality show *The Biggest Loser.* On the television program, which challenges overweight people to lose big pounds, contestants living on a secluded ranch are responsible for preparing all of their own meals from healthy, fresh ingredients. "The kitchen is a big part of their training," says Harper. "Prior to coming on the show, many of the contestants would eat most of their meals at restaurants."

RULE #4: DROP CARBS. ADD PROTEIN

On the Belly Off! Diet meal plan, it is crucial to eliminate or cut way back on cakes, cookies, candy, soda, fruit juice, white bread, pasta, potatoes, sugary breakfast cereals, and anything that has high fructose corn syrup in it, like fruit juices and jarred spaghetti sauce. All of these are fast-absorbing carbohydrates, the foods that spike blood sugar, instigate cravings, and help fat set up residence in the belly region. Remember, nearly 100 percent of the *Men's Health* Belly Off! Club guys used this strategy to lose their guts. And dozens of studies support the case that restricting carbohydrates forces your body to burn fat. If you're not sure about a product, simply check the ingredient list: Skip those that contain sugar—often listed as sucrose, high fructose corn syrup, or cane syrup—and refined flour, which likely is any flour that doesn't start with the word "whole" (as in whole wheat).

IT WORKS FOR ME

"Get a partner. Find someone who's as motivated as you are. He can help you on days you don't want to go, and you can help him, too."

—J.K. Crews, Glenville, GA, who lost 115 pounds

CHEAT SHEET
How to Speed Read a Food Label

Reading food labels is easy if you know how to cut through the clutter and find the important info. Here's your four-point cheat sheet. Use it when comparing nutrition facts labels to make the healthiest choice between similar products.

LOOK FOR . . .

1. TRANS FATS

Zero is best. Check the ingredients list for "partially hydrogenated," as you see in this label, "interesterified," or "stearate-rich" oils. If you find them, don't buy. Find another product.

2. FIBER

More is better. Keeps you fuller longer. Reduces cholesterol.

3. SUGARS

Less is better. Look for the total carbohydrate line. Then read down to the breakout for sugars. When choosing between two similar products, go for the one that has fewer grams of sugar. This is the stuff that can spike your blood sugar and trigger an insulin rush. Still a close call when comparing two products? Then check out 4.

4. NUMBER OF INGREDIENTS

Fewer is better. The product contains more of the stuff found at the top of the list than at the bottom. Here you can see that this product, a breakfast cereal, is mostly sugar. As a general rule, foods with the least number of ingredients will be better for you.

Nutrition Facts

Serving Size 1 Cup (32g/1.1 oz.)
Servings Per Container About 10

Amount Per Serving	Cereal	Cereal with 1/2 Cup Vitamins A&D Fat Free Milk
Calories	120	160
Calories from Fat	10	10

	% Daily Value**	
Total Fat 1g*	**2%**	**2%**
Saturated Fat 0.5g	**3%**	**3%**
Trans Fat 0g		
Cholesterol 0mg	**0%**	**0%**
Sodium 150mg	**6%**	**9%**
Potassium 35mg	**1%**	**7%**
Total Carbohydrate 28g	**9%**	**11%**
Dietary Fiber 1g	**4%**	**4%**
Sugars 15g		
Other Carbohydrate 12g		
Protein 1g		

Vitamin A	10%	15%
Vitamin C	25%	25%
Calcium	0%	15%
Iron	25%	25%
Vitamin D	10%	25%
Thiamin	25%	30%
Riboflavin	25%	35%
Niacin	25%	25%
Vitamin B$_6$	25%	25%
Folic Acid	25%	25%
Vitamin B$_{12}$	25%	35%
Phosphorus	2%	15%
Zinc	10%	15%

* Amount in cereal. One half cup of fat free milk contributes an additional 40 calories, 65mg sodium, 6g total carbohydrates (6g sugars), and 4g protein.
**Percent Daily Values are based on a 2,000 calorie diet. Your daily values may be higher or lower depending on your calorie needs:

	Calories	2,000	2,500
Total Fat	Less than	65g	80g
Saturated Fat	Less than	20g	25g
Cholesterol	Less than	300mg	300mg
Sodium	Less than	2,400mg	2,400mg
Potassium		3,500mg	3,500mg
Total Carbohydrate		300g	375g
Dietary Fiber		25g	30g

Calories per gram: Fat 9 • Carbohydrate 4 • Protein 4

INGREDIENTS: SUGAR; CORN FLOUR; WHEAT FLOUR; OAT FLOUR; PARTIALLY HYDROGENATED VEGETABLE OIL (ONE OR MORE OF: COCONUT, COTTONSEED, AND SOYBEAN); SALT; SODIUM ASCORBATE AND ASCORBIC ACID (VITAMIN C); NIACINAMIDE; REDUCED IRON; NATURAL ORANGE, LEMON, CHERRY, RASPBERRY, BLUEBERRY, LIME, AND OTHER NATURAL FLAVORS; RED #40; BLUE #2; ZINC OXIDE; YELLOW #6; TURMERIC COLOR; PYRIDOXINE HYDROCHLORIDE (VITAMIN B$_6$); BLUE #1; RIBOFLAVIN (VITAMIN B$_2$); THIAMIN HYDROCHLORIDE (VITAMIN B$_1$); ANNATTO COLOR; VITAMIN A PALMITATE; BHT (PRESERVATIVE); FOLIC ACID; VITAMIN B$_{12}$; VITAMIN D.

Recently, a study at the University of California at Davis offered evidence to explain how cutting down on carbs may trigger weight loss. Researchers there found that keeping carbs to less than 40 percent of your total daily calories actually deactivates a gene that produces triglycerides—the blood fats that collect as body fat.

Putting this fat-busting DNA modification to work is not hard or complicated. *You should automatically achieve it just by following the basic guidelines and recipes in this book.* Protein foods like steak, chicken, pork, and seafood all have *zero* carbs. Whole fruit has fewer than juice (a cup of grapes has 16 grams of carbs; a cup of grape juice, 36). Green and red vegetables are low in carbs—a whole cup of cooked carrots or broccoli has about 6 grams. French fries are loaded—a medium portion has 47, and the super size has 77. A large chocolate chip cookie has 59 grams, and if you wash it down with a 20-ounce Coke, you're getting another 60!

Slow-burning *complex carbohydrates* are essential to good health. Replace the *fast-burning* carbs found in highly processed foods in your diet with vegetables and whole fruits, whole-grain bread, brown rice, and whole-wheat pasta. These high-volume foods are rich in fiber, "the best thing you can eat when you are trying to lose weight," says Gay Riley, a registered dietitian in Dallas, Texas. Fiber binds with other foods to help hustle calories out of the body and because they slow your rate of digestion, they keep you feeling full longer and reduce cravings for more food, especially sugary foods.

SUPERSHOT
Don't Inhale
Your Dinner

You can decrease your calorie consumption by 10 percent simply by slowing down between bites and taking a few breaths, according to a study at the University of Rhode Island.

TRY TO GET 5 GRAMS OF FIBER AT EVERY MEAL. THE FOLLOWING FOODS HAVE AT LEAST THAT MUCH:

- 1 cup of any breakfast cereal with "bran" in the name

- 1 cup of cooked pinto, black, kidney, or navy beans

- A large apple or two medium pears

FOODS THAT HAVE 2 TO 4 GRAMS OF DIETARY FIBER:

- 1 cup of any fruit that ends in "berry"

- A handful of almonds, peanuts, cashews, or sunflower seeds

- 1 cup of cooked broccoli, carrots, cauliflower, green beans, spinach, or asparagus

- 1 cup of cooked whole-wheat pasta or brown rice

- Two slices of whole-wheat bread

If you need a little extra help getting more fiber into your stomach, try this: Mix a tablespoon of Metamucil in a glass of water and drink it about 5 minutes before you eat a meal. (Don't worry; the new formulation isn't gloppy like the old stuff, and it's available in an orange flavor.) The psyllium fiber in Metamucil will start to fill you up so you may eat less. In addition, the fiber will bind with the food you eat, creating a gooey slurry that will slow down digestion, even if you ate some fast-digesting starch. In essence, that fiber drink will lower the glycemic load of your meal!

In addition to fiber, the Belly Off! Diet also encourages you to eat some protein and fat with every meal. Fat because it is satiating. It adds satisfying flavor to foods, and it makes you feel as if you ate something substantial. Protein because it is your strongest ally in the war against a big belly. Here are some reasons why:

- Protein makes you feel full quicker and it takes about 2 hours longer than carbs to digest, so you won't get hungry as soon.

- It takes more energy for your body to digest protein than it does for it to digest carbohydrates or fat. "Protein burns hotter than other food sources," says Mark Hyman, MD, author of *Ultrametabolism*. So the more protein you eat, the more calories you'll burn in the process of digestion. A British study found that people who increased the percentage of calories from protein in their meals burned 71 more calories per day than people on low-protein diets. (That amounts to 7.4 pounds of body-weight lost per year.)

- Protein accelerates muscle growth and speeds your recovery after vigorous exercise by helping to rebuild stressed muscle fibers.

How much protein you should get depends upon your level of activity. The USDA's Recommended Dietary Allowance (RDA) for protein is 0.37 gram per pound of bodyweight per day. But if you're running or doing resistance exercises, you probably need 0.45 gram or more per pound, or about 90 grams of protein per day for a 200-pound man.

Terrific sources of protein are lean meats and fish and other animal products, such as eggs, milk, and cheese. Four ounces of chicken breast, for example, contains about 32 grams of protein. You can also get your protein from beans, lentils, nuts, and seeds. A half cup of black beans delivers about 8 grams.

RULE #5: AVOID ALCOHOL

If you are a guy who enjoys a couple of beers every night, some wine with dinner, and maybe margaritas on the weekends, cutting out alcohol will give you an enormous head start on shedding pounds and belly fat. Abstain for a month, and you'll be convinced. Alcohol stops your body from burning fat, and depending upon what you drink (beer or cocktails made with sugary mixers), that beverage can be loaded with empty carbohydrates. Cutting booze of all types for just 4 weeks is the best way to start controlling your sugar intake. It won't be forever. Just 4 weeks. You can do it.

THE GLOSSARY OF FAT

Let's spend a few moments chewing the fat. Two things immediately come to mind when I think of fat: the roll of it creeping over my belt, which I loathe, and a certain Hungarian peasant food called *szalonna,* which I love. Szalonna is a chunk of smoked pork fat speared on a green stick and roasted over fruitwood coals until it drips smoky, bacony, delicious grease. You press the hot drippings into a slice of rye bread sprinkled with paprika, top it with raw onion and cucumber slices, and eat. Szalonna may be the Antichrist to a cardiologist, but, by God, it's good—in minimal quantities. I eat it once—and only once—a year at our family's Hungarian Hoedown family reunion. Eat enough of this stuff, and you might as well point a pistol toward your heart and pull the trigger.

Doctors and nutritionists have been warning us about the dangers of a diet high in fats for years. An entire health-products industry has sprouted from the idea that fat equals poison. Yet while government statistics show that our fat consumption has been dropping, the number of fat Americans has been rising.

One reason, many experts agree, is that we are eating many more calories than ever before, thanks to fat-free foods. Less fat equals less guilt equals more eating. Some doctors have even suggested that if we weren't so anal about eating fat, we'd all be a lot thinner.

While being less vigilant about dietary fat is an appealing notion it is still important to be cognizant of the total amount of fat that you eat and remember that calories still matter. Even more important is understanding the type of fat that you eat. Here's a primer.

Saturated fats: You find them mainly in meats, butter, cheese, eggs, shortening, and tropical oils. Saturated fats are typically solid at room temperature. So if you can carve it into a swan, you can be sure that swan is saturated. Some saturated fats raise your low-density lipoprotein (LDL) or "bad" cholesterol,

FIT FACT

British researchers found that men who wore pedometers and logged their daily steps in a journal boosted their activity levels by 16 percent.

and increase your risk of heart disease and stroke. But a growing number of researchers believe the real culprit is consuming too many calories and overeating carbohydrates. In fact, some studies show that when people replace carbohydrates in their diet with fat—saturated or unsaturated—the number of the most dangerous LDL particles actually decreases. The message from these researchers is not to gorge on butter and bacon, but that there's no scientific evidence to suggest that natural foods containing saturated fat shouldn't be a part of a healthy diet. The American Heart Association recommends that a 40-year-old man of average height and weighing about 180 limit himself to about 200 calories of saturated fats per day. If you are not overweight, you don't smoke, you exercise regularly and you eat a healthy diet, then you probably don't have to worry much about going over that limit.

Trans fat: It's in stick margarine, crackers, cookies, cakes, and corn dogs. Expect to find it in anything that's deep fried. In processed foods, a trans fat is created when hydrogen is added to vegetable oil to keep it "stable" for frying (unstable oil makes food taste bad) and to prevent it from going rancid. It's what makes a half-eaten Twinkie you just found under your couch look as new as it did when your nephew hid it there a year and a half ago.

Trans fats are, for the most part, manufactured fats. In order to remove cholesterol from their products, makers of processed foods have been replacing saturated fats (such as lard and beef tallow) with hydrogenated vegetable oils. They take vegetable oil, heat it to high temperatures, and pump in hydrogen, which bonds with the oil molecules to create a new form of fat that stays solid at room temperature. This is ideal for makers of cookies, cakes, muffins, waffles, candy bars, and fish sticks, who need oil in a solid form to make their products taste good and look appealing. The words "hydrogenated" or "partially hydrogenated" on the ingredients list will tip you off to the trans fats.

Trans fat should be aggressively avoided because of its unhealthy effect on your cholesterol levels—increasing LDL cholesterol and lowering the "good" high-density lipoprotein (HDL) cholesterol. Trans fat has also been shown increase triglycerides and it appears to damage cells lining blood vessels, leading to inflammation.

Though the dangers of trans fat have been highly publicized, that message seems to have been lost on the carnival crowd. We hear that funnel cakes are being replaced by a new rage on the midway: batter-dipped, deep-fried Oreo cookies.

Monounsaturated fats: You'll find these in olive, canola, and peanut oils. Studies show that these fats can also help you *burn* fat. And because they're digested slowly, they make you feel fuller longer. These fats are also considered "heart healthy," because they either have no effect on cholesterol levels or, in the form of oleic acid, lower LDL cholesterol without affecting HDL cholesterol. But that's no green light to sponge up a bowl of olive oil with a loaf of crusty Italian bread. Only 15 percent of your daily fat calories should come from these fats.

Polyunsaturated fats: These show up in corn, safflower, soybean, and sunflower oils. Unlike monos, polys lower both LDL and HDL. But animal research has shown that a type of polyunsaturated fat called conjugated linoleic acid, CLA for short, found in certain meats and dairy products, may have strong health benefits—including reducing abdominal fat, protecting against heart disease and diabetes, and inhibiting the growth of prostate cancer cells.

Essential fatty acids: Omega-6 and omega-3 fatty acids are the two basic ones; they fall under the polyunsaturated fats umbrella. We get more omega-6s than we need from cooking oils, meat, eggs, and dairy products, but not nearly enough omega-3s, which are found in certain types of fish and in walnuts, flaxseed, and green leafy vegetables. Focus on

REAL GUYS—REAL RESULTS

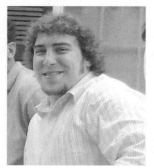

BEFORE:
290
POUNDS

AFTER:
210
POUNDS

"I was eating myself to death."

VITALS: **Dan Sizelove, 24, Brick, NJ**
OCCUPATION: **Marketing coordinator**
HEIGHT: **6'1"**
LESSON LEARNED: **Believing in your ability to stay on track is essential.**

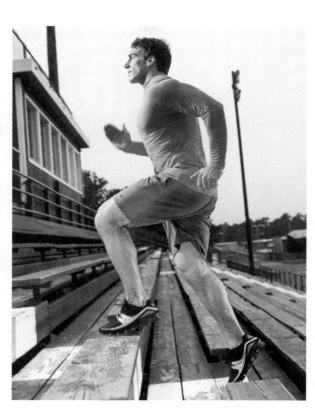

As a defensive lineman in college, Sizelove followed a hardcore lifting routine that helped him pack on muscle. But a lack of cardio exercise, coupled with poor food choices and plenty of late-night boozing, added 65 pounds of fat to his once-athletic frame. "I blamed my weight gain on being a lineman, but that was really just a scapegoat," Sizelove says.

THE TURNING POINT
With no more football to turn to, Sizelove set his sights on running a 5-K, but his weight was holding him back and he felt a void in his life from being inactive. He decided that a lifestyle change was necessary, so he hit the gym, focusing first on interval training to burn off blubber. Eventually, he added weight training and watched more pounds fall off.

LIFE IN THE FIT LANE
Sizelove lifts weights four times a week, runs frequently, and bikes to work as often as he can. Having the freedom to map out his own workouts instead of mindlessly following a coach's instructions has boosted his motivation as well. Sizelove now eats more protein, such as chicken and fish, and has reined in his college habit of snacking on chips

and pretzels late at night.

THE REWARD
Old friends are astonished when they see Sizelove's new physique, and his energy level has skyrocketed. "I don't even need coffee to wake up anymore," he says. He already one-upped that 5-K goal by running a second one.

SIZELOVE'S BEST BELLY OFF! TIPS
•Stop counting calories. Adding up every bite is

demoralizing and only reminds you of the foods you can't have.
●Take things day by day, and accept the fact that your body won't transform itself overnight.
●Break through plateaus. A stall in weight loss is frustrating, but even a small change—like running instead of biking one day a week—can be the push you need.

getting more omega-3s. The richest sources are oily fish like sardines, mackerel, tuna, and salmon. But if you don't like fish, you can take a fish-oil supplement. Some of these liquids and oil-filled capsules can make you belch like a pelican. So look for the new formulations available at health food stores that attempt to eliminate the low-tide aftertaste.

Omega-3s are important because they appear to slow the body's production of prostaglandins—chemical compounds that can cause excessive blood clotting, which can lead to heart attacks. In addition, omega-3s are thought to influence your metabolism, determining whether you burn calories or store them as fat, by altering levels of a hormone called leptin in your body. Studies have found a correlation between

A FINE KETTLE OF FISH
Top Seafoods for Omega-3s

The average American man eats about 15 pounds of fish a year. Most of that comes in the form of fried shrimp, fried fish sticks, and fried fillets on a bun with tartar sauce—all loaded with fat, salt, and calories. You can do much better by choosing fish that's high in omega-3 fats and having it steamed, grilled, broiled, baked, or poached. Here are the specifications on the best of the best seafoods, according to the Cleveland Clinic.

FISH*	OMEGA-3 CONTENT
Herring	1.9 g
Sardines	1.5 g
Bluefin tuna	1.5 g
Atlantic mackerel	1.5 g
Salmon	1.0 g
Swordfish	0.9 g
Sea bass	0.65 g
Tuna (white meat), canned	0.5 g
Flounder	0.4 g
Jumbo shrimp (6 pieces)	0.15 g
Lobster	0.15 g

* All 3-ounce servings.

low levels of leptin and a faster metabolism. In research at the University of South Australia's Nutritional Physiology Research Centre, overweight men were assigned to one of two groups: One group ate tuna or took fish oil and did aerobic exercise; the other group took sunflower oil and also exercised. At the end of 12 weeks, the exercisers who consumed omega-3s reduced their body fat and improved their metabolic and cardiovascular health. The sunflower oil sippers experienced no such benefit, but their breath smelled a whole lot better.

Now on to seeds and nuts. You know what a walnut is, so let me give a quick shout out to flaxseed, a powerful food that until recently has gotten very little press. This stuff, which looks like shiny brown sesame seeds, is packed with omega-3s plus cholesterol-fighting fiber. When you can't get a hold of some fish to eat, flaxseeds are an easy way to get your omega-3s. You can sprinkle them on breakfast cereal, toss them into soups and stews, even use them in spaghetti with tomato sauce. They've got a nice nutty flavor, so they're tasty mixed into yogurt or sprinkled on top of ice cream. Buy a bag at the health food store to keep on hand; they're available whole or ground. You might also find flaxseed at your supermarket as grocers become hip to this trendy seed.

THE 7-DAY QUICK-START GUIDE

Every Tool You Need to Lose Weight in a Week

THINK BACK TO WHEN you were a teenager sleeping until noon on a Saturday after a late night. Did your dad ever grab the edge of the mattress and flip you out of bed to get you moving? Mine did. And he'd often hand me a sheet of paper with a list of the day's chores. Don't get me wrong. Dad's a sweet guy who taught me more about hard work, integrity, and the importance of having a higher purpose in your life than any book or class ever did. In hindsight, I'm grateful that he got me in gear. How else would I have learned how to clean the carburetor on a lawnmower, fix leaky gutters, lay brick, and paint trim? A kick in the pants is a good thing now and then, even if you're not a teenager anymore. Having a plan of action is even better.

So, to make the Belly Off! Diet easy to incorporate into your life, we've listed the steps you'll need to take during this first week. You don't have to think. Just follow along. And you'll get the picture by Friday.

Step 1. With your food diary in hand, clean out your refrigerator and pantry, paying particular attention to the bad stuff your diary identified. Dump any pastas, cereals, or breads that aren't 100 percent whole wheat, and any non-diet soda.

Step 2. Copy Week 1 Shopping List at right, take it to the grocery store, and stock up. Everything you need to eat for the first week is on the shopping list. Follow the week's meal plan to the letter. (Use the recipes and cooking instructions where needed.) Don't worry. You're going to love this food. It's guy food. It tastes great. It's designed to automatically control calories, saturated fat, and carbs, while energizing your body with metabolism-revving fuel. Eating this way for just 1 week will eliminate any guesswork until you realize the logic of the diet and you can tailor your own weekly meal plans to your specific tastes later on.

Step 3. Follow the exercise schedule outlined on page 61. The descriptions of the workouts and exercises can be found in Chapter 5. By knowing how you are going to exercise every day and what you're going to eat, you'll be more likely to make this quick-start a ritual.

HOW TO EAT

Start by hunting and gathering at your local supermarket. You'll note in the shopping list the occasional brand name product. These are foods we've had some personal experience with, which we can recommend as exceptional. Perhaps your grocer stocks them. If this shopping list looks extra long, well, there's a reason for that. It includes a lot of new food items, condiments, and other staples to stock your pantry with and use for weeks to come. And it's likely that

(continued on page 60)

WEEK 1 SHOPPING LIST

DAIRY

Eggland's Best eggs (these contain heart-healthy omega-3 fats) hard cheese	low-fat chocolate milk low-fat string cheese low-fat vanilla ice cream low-fat yogurt	mozzarella cheese 1% or fat-free milk pepper Jack cheese	reduced-fat Cheddar cheese Swiss cheese slices reduced-fat sour cream

FRUITS AND VEGETABLES

apples asparagus avocado baby carrots bananas basil leaves blueberries broccoli	cantaloupe celery cilantro corn dates grape tomatoes green leaf lettuce mushrooms	orange, red, and green peppers oranges pears raisins red grapes red onions romaine lettuce	scallions sprouts strawberries tomatoes yellow onions zucchini

BREAD, CEREAL, PASTA

couscous Kashi GoLean high-protein cereal Kellogg's All-Bran cereal oatmeal (steel cut)	Pepperidge Farm Whole Grain Double Fiber 100% Whole Wheat Bread	whole-wheat hamburger buns whole-wheat pasta	whole-wheat pizza crust whole-wheat tortillas

BEANS, NUTS, RICE

brown rice canned black beans	canned pinto beans	canned red kidney beans	raw almonds

MEATS AND FISH

Canadian bacon extra-lean ground beef ground turkey breast	nitrate-free turkey bacon salmon fillet	skinless, boneless chicken breast	sliced roast turkey breast deli meat

OTHER

Arrowhead Mills Creamy Almond Butter blue corn tortilla chips Caesar salad dressing canned diced tomatoes canned low-salt whole tomatoes	canned shrimp canned sliced jalapenos canned tomato paste and tomato sauce canned vegetarian barbecued beans chicken noodle soup	chipotle salsa cranberry juice cocktail garlic cloves garlic-flavored hummus Honest Tea Organic Honey Green Tea mint leaves	nonstick cooking spray orange juice with calcium and pulp popcorn roasted red pepper strips trail mix

CONDIMENTS, SPICES, AND OTHER USEFUL STUFF
TO STOCK UP ON IF YOU DON'T ALREADY HAVE THEM

blueberry or raspberry preserves brown sugar cayenne pepper coffee Crazy Richard's 100% Natural Chunky peanut butter Dijon mustard extra-virgin olive oil	flaxseeds (available at health food stores) garlic bulbs ground black pepper green and black tea bags Hellmann's Olive Oil Mayonnaise Dressing Italian seasoning ketchup lemon juice	low-fat cream cheese low-sodium soy sauce olives, Greek Kalamata or Italian Cerignola peanut butter red pepper flakes reduced-fat mayonnaise rice wine vinegar salsa sea salt	sesame flakes sesame oil sesame seeds sun-dried tomatoes sun-dried tomato pesto Tabasco sauce taco seasoning Worcestershire sauce

YOUR REAL MEAL MENU FOR WEEK 1

	Monday	Tuesday	Wednesday
6:30 A.M. **BREAKFAST**	Scrambled eggs made with 3 eggs (1 yolk, 2 whites) 2 slices turkey bacon 1 slice whole-wheat toast with 1 Tbsp of almond or peanut butter 1 piece of fruit Coffee, black (optional) 8 oz cold water	1 bowl of bran cereal with fat-free milk 1 banana with almond butter Coffee, tea, or orange juice cut with water	Huevos Rancheros Wrap (recipe page 179) with Canadian bacon Coffee or tea 8 oz cold water
10 A.M. **MORNING SNACK**	1 pear 1 stick of low-fat string cheese 8 oz cold water	Celery sticks filled with cream cheese and chopped olives spread	5 strawberries 1 cup low-fat yogurt 8 oz cold water
1:30 P.M. **LUNCH**	Chicken Caesar Salad (no croutons) 2 Tbsp Caesar Salad Dressing 8 oz unsweetened iced tea or water	Mediterranean Wrap (recipe page 184) 1 apple Honest Tea Green Tea	Peanut butter and preserves sandwich Low-fat chocolate milk
4 P.M. **AFTERNOON SNACK**	1 oz dates 1 oz almonds 8 oz cold water or diet soda	1 cup berries 1 oz hard cheese	1 handful of raw almonds String cheese Unsweetened iced tea
7 P.M. **DINNER**	1 cup chicken noodle soup Three-Alarm Sloppy Joes (recipe page 190) ½ cup cole slaw 15 red grapes 8 oz cold water or green tea	Grilled chicken breast, Grilled Asparagus (recipe page 192), couscous Fat-free milk, water, or unsweetened iced tea	Men's Health One-Pot Turkey Chili (recipe page 174) Unsweetened iced tea Cantaloupe slices
9 P.M. **EVENING SNACK (OPTIONAL)**	1 cup air-popped popcorn	Low-fat ice cream	15 frozen red grapes

Thursday	Friday	Saturday	Sunday
Almond butter and raspberry preserves sandwich on whole-wheat bread 1 medium apple Coffee, fat-free milk, or orange juice 8 oz cold water	1 bowl of Kashi GoLean high-protein cereal 2 slices cantaloupe Coffee, tea, or orange juice	Easy, Cheesy Breakfast Burrito (recipe page 181) 1/2 cup blueberries Coffee, tea, or orange juice 8 oz cold water	Ham, onion, peppers, and mushroom egg white omelet Orange juice (cut in half with water) 1 slice whole-wheat toast (with a pat of butter) 2 slices cantaloupe Coffee or tea
Cheese wedges 1/2 cup blueberries	1 oz almonds 1 apple	Almond butter on a banana	1 apple with 1 Tbsp almond butter
Leftover turkey chili 1/2 cup strawberries Diet soda	Turkey bacon, lettuce, and tomato sandwich on whole-wheat toast with low-fat mayonnaise	Chipotle Turkey Burgers (recipe page 206) Corn and black bean salad Iced green tea	Turkey bacon, lettuce, and tomato sandwich on whole-wheat toast with low-fat mayonnaise
Raw baby carrots 1 oz hummus 8 oz cold water	Low-fat cheese stick 2 handfuls of trail mix	Raw baby carrots 1 oz hummus	Celery sticks with low-fat cream cheese and olive spread
Grilled salmon Brown rice Steamed broccoli Green salad Unsweetened iced tea Red grapes	Belly Off! Pizza with The Works (recipe page 187) Garden salad Unsweetened iced tea	Eat-It-Cold Shrimp and Pasta Salad (recipe page 186) 6 oz cranberry juice cocktail cut with about 2 oz water Orange wedges	Taco Salad (recipe page 194) Black beans Brown rice Iced tea
2 oz trail mix 1 cup low-fat chocolate milk	Low-fat vanilla ice cream	1/2 cup low-fat vanilla ice cream	2 oz trail mix 1 cup low-fat chocolate milk

SUPERSHOT
Soup Up
Your Broth

Toss ½ cup of
chickpeas into a pot
of your favorite
soup. They'll take
on the flavor of the
soup and tack 6
grams of fiber onto
your bottom line.

you have some of this stuff, like peanut butter and
Tabasco sauce, already on hand.

Still, you may find yourself paying more at the
grocery store when using this list because better
foods and fresh meats and vegetables tend to cost
more than processed and packaged foods. But eating
more meals at home and fewer at restaurants will
ultimately save you money. And if you are smart
about using leftovers, these recipes can save you time
as well.

STRATEGIC SNACKING
Keep Hunger at Bay with These Combinations

There's a simple science to snacking on the
Belly Off! Diet, and it goes like this:

•Snack frequently before your blood sugar
drops, about 3 hours after you last ate a meal.
•Combine carbohydrates with protein or dairy
to fend off the belly grumbles of hunger and
keep blood sugar stable.

•Keep healthy snacks within reach, as in a
drawer in your office at work. If you have to hunt
for them, you're more likely to grab the wrong
kind. Plan ahead with the suggestions below. And
consider bringing dinner leftovers for a quick
snack. Roll a leftover piece of chicken breast in a
tortilla with a spoonful of salsa. You're done.
Here are some other suggested combos:

CARBOHYDRATE	+	PROTEIN OR DAIRY
5 strawberries	+	1 cup low-fat yogurt
Raw baby carrots	+	1 oz hummus
1 oz dates	+	1 oz almonds
1 medium apple	+	1 Tbsp peanut butter, 1 cup 1% milk
2 oz trail mix	+	1 cup low-fat chocolate milk
Celery sticks	+	Cream cheese
Whole-wheat tortilla	+	2 slices turkey breast and 1 slice Swiss cheese
1 pear	+	1 stick of low-fat string cheese
1 cup berries	+	1 oz hard cheese

HOW TO EXERCISE

THE BELLY OFF! WORKOUT SCHEDULE

MONDAY	TUESDAY	WEDNESDAY	THURSDAY	FRIDAY	SATURDAY	SUNDAY
2-Minute Drill	2-Minute Drill	2-Minute Drill	2-Minute Drill	2-Minute Drill	2-Minute Drill	Rest
Bodyweight 100/200	Cardio Intervals	Bodyweight 100/200	Cardio Intervals	Bodyweight 100/200	Cardio Intervals	

THE SECRET: START EACH DAY WITH THE BELLY OFF! 2-MINUTE DRILL

Why do you try to schedule a doctor's visit for the first appointment of the day? To get in and out fast and avoid the waiting-room time suck (and those blue-haired ladies). Why is it best to take the first flight out in the morning? Because airport delays are more likely as the day progresses. For the same reason, you want to get some exercise in at the start of the day because commitments, interruptions, and fires at work can destroy your best-laid plans to exercise.

For me, morning is the only time of day that I can control. That's why I love the 2-Minute Drill designed by personal trainer David Jack, the guy you see in the workout photographs. Do it as soon as you get up. Don't even bother changing into workout clothes. It's just eight calisthenics that take just 2 minutes. I knock mine out while I'm waiting for the coffee to brew.

The Belly Off! 2-Minute Drill is a brilliant beginning to your day because it jump-starts your metabolism, revving it higher to start burning fat all day. Exercise in the morning also helps to wake you up, bringing oxygen into your brain to shed the cobwebs of sleep and triggering your body to release endorphins, feel-good hormones, into your bloodstream. Plus, it starts your day on a positive note. Even if the rest of my day is a disaster, even if I can't squeeze in

IT WORKS FOR ME

"Add flavor to your foods (hot sauce, cracked black pepper, and spices). It's easier to skimp on calories if you satisfy your taste buds."

—Ryan Hubers, Lake Forest, CA, who lost 165 pounds

Heavy guys sometimes have trouble running because of the stress their weight puts on their knees. If you are one of them, you can reduce your risk of injury and still get a great workout by going for a walk instead of a joint-pounding jog. A new study at A.T. Still University found that walking 3 mph on a treadmill set at an incline can be as challenging as running on a flat surface. The researchers say walking on an incline of 6, 9, 12, and 15 percent at 3 mph is equal to running flat at speeds of 4, 5, 6, and 7 mph respectively.

my regular workout, I'll knock out a circuit of three more 2-minute drills later on, and I'm at least able to say I've broken a sweat for 8 minutes today.

So make the 2-Minute Drill part of your morning routine. In a matter of weeks, it'll become so rote, it'll seem awkward to skip, like walking out the door without brushing your teeth. Perform the following eight-calisthenic circuit at a work effort of 6 to 7 on a scale of 1 to 10. Do each exercise for 15 seconds, then move immediately to the next until you have done all eight in just 2 minutes.

The beauty of the 2-Minute Drill is that you can do it anywhere—on a business trip, in your office, or waiting in line for Jonas Brothers tickets for your 12-year-old.

THE BELLY OFF! 2-MINUTE DRILL

8 MOVES EVERY MORNING

(Complete as many reps as you can of each exercise during each 15-second time slot.)

Jumping Jacks	15 seconds
Prisoner Squats	15 seconds
High Knee Skips	15 seconds
Side-to-Side Hops	15 seconds
Pushups	15 seconds
Crunches	15 seconds
Mountain Climbers	15 seconds
Bodyweight Thrusters	15 seconds

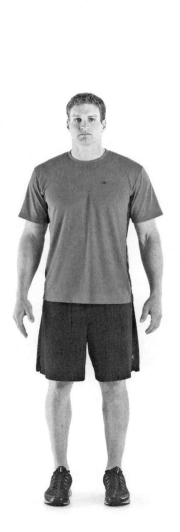
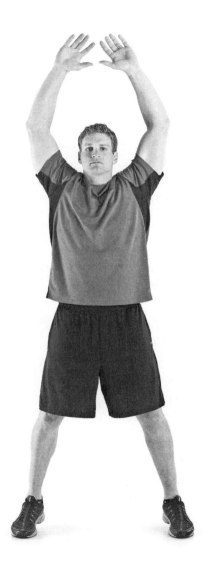

1. JUMPING JACKS (15 SECONDS)

Just like you remember from gym class. Start with your feet hip-width apart and hands at your sides. Simultaneously raise your arms above your head and jump up so you can spread your feet shoulder-width apart. Then jump again to lower your arms and bring your feet together. Repeat.

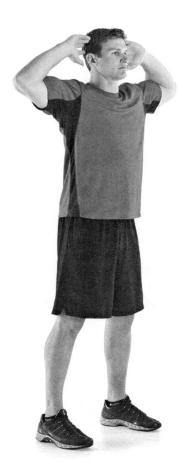
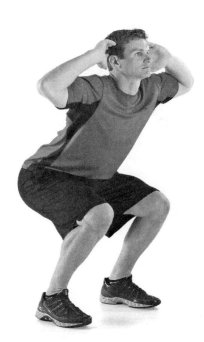

2. PRISONER SQUATS (15 SECONDS)

Stand with your fingertips behind your ears, your chest out, elbows back, and feet shoulder-width apart. Sit back at your hips and bend your knees to lower your body as far as you can without losing the natural arch of your spine. Squeeze your gluteals and push yourself back to the starting position.

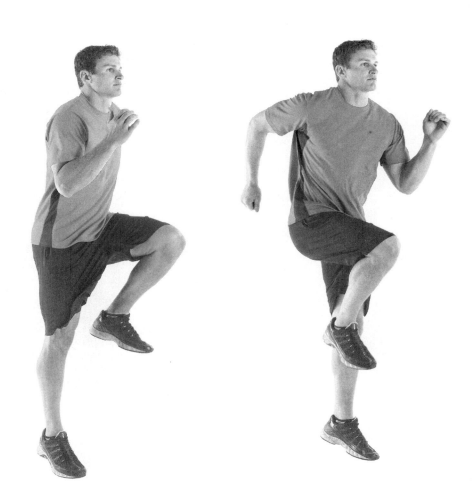

3. HIGH KNEE SKIPS (15 SECONDS)

Keeping your upper body straight, drive a knee as high up and out as you can, alternating knees while skipping. As you drive each knee up, swing your opposite hand upward to get as much vertical lift as possible. For a smoother rhythm, add a hop on the downward step.

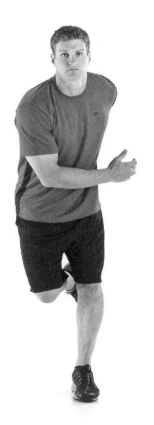
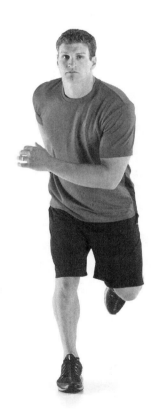

4. SIDE-TO-SIDE HOPS (15 SECONDS)

Starting with feet together, push off with your right foot to hop laterally to the left about 3 feet. Land on your left foot and follow with your right. Hop back, this time pushing off with your left foot. Repeat.

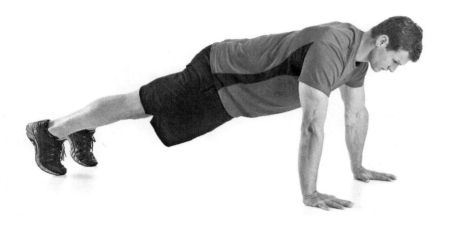

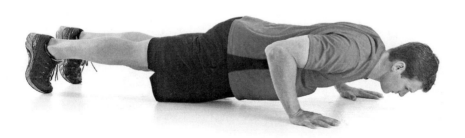

5. PUSHUPS (15 SECONDS)

With hands on the floor, shoulder-width apart, and back straight, lower yourself to touch your chest to the floor—you know the drill. But here's a tip: Keep your abdominal muscles pulled in and taut. Think of drawing your belly button toward your spine. This does two things: It helps you burn more calories because you are engaging more muscle fibers and it will help you maintain proper form.

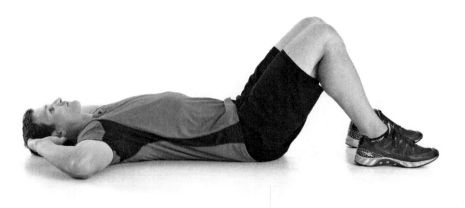

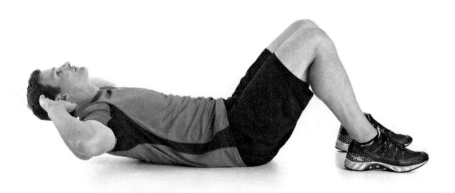

6. CRUNCHES (15 SECONDS)

Lie on your back with knees bent and feet flat on the floor. Put your hands behind your head so that your fingertips brush your ears. Don't grab your head; that'll put strain on your neck. Keeping your neck in alignment with your straight back, use your abs to lift your shoulders off the floor a few inches, no more. Release back down and repeat.

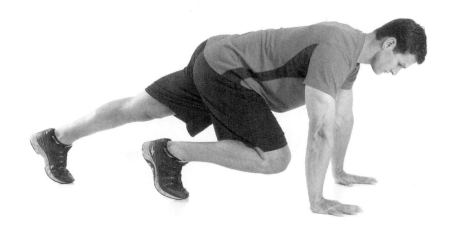

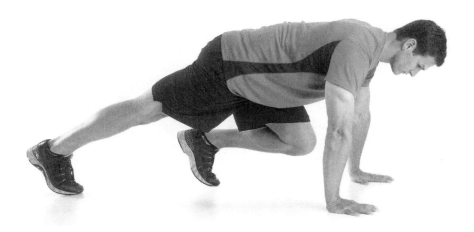

7. MOUNTAIN CLIMBERS (15 SECONDS)

Start in a pushup position with your shoulders directly over your hands. Keeping your head in line with your body, bring your right knee to your chest. As you straighten the right leg back to the starting position, bring your left knee to your chest. Keep your weight on the balls of your feet. As quickly as possible, "climb," alternating your legs back and forth.

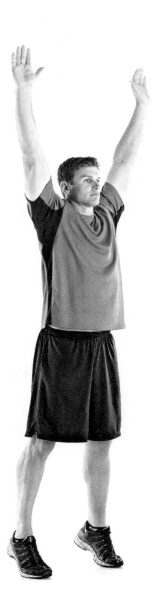

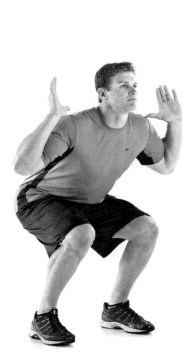

8. BODYWEIGHT THRUSTERS (15 SECONDS)

Keeping your back straight and hands at your shoulders as if you were holding a barbell, bend at the knees into a squat, then explosively drive your legs straight while extending your arms above your head. That's 1 rep.

WHAT TO DO IF YOU FIND THE 2-MINUTE DRILL TOO DIFFICULT

The Belly Off! 2-Minute Drill will get anyone huffing and puffing. It's a good, quick morning jump start for most people. But it may not be for everyone. If you are heavy or have been sedentary for a long period of time, or even if you find one of the eight exercises painful or too difficult, you are free to change the drill to suit your situation. This drill isn't set in stone; it's highly customizable. Remember: The purpose of the 2-Minute Drill is to get your body moving in the morning to kick-start your metabolism for the day. And just about any series of calisthenics will do that. Heck, you might want to start out by climbing up and down your basement stairs for 2 minutes. Or you might design your own 2-Minute Drill with your favorite exercises.

To mix things up, I've done a 2-Minute Drill of rope jumping, pushups, and crunches. A friend of mine, who was recovering from knee surgery, customized his morning routine to focus on simple upper-body exercises so he wouldn't have to stress his knee. He did wall pumps (basically pushups against a wall, performed while standing); military presses and curls holding cans of baked beans; seated torso rotations; and crunches. One Belly Off! Club Member uses his tai chi practice as his 2-Minute Drill. The point is to do what works for you. For 2 minutes every morning.

FIT FACT

15

Percentage by which a person's productivity rises on an exercise day, according to British researchers

GET BACK IN SHAPE FAST WITH INTERVALS

We interrupt this workout for a brief public service announcement: It's always a good idea to see your physician for a checkup before starting an exercise program and especially after a layoff from exercise of any significant period of time. Just to be safe. Please do it for yourself.

Okay, back to sweating. If you've been away from exercise, the best strategy is to lose some fat first, *then* add muscle. Do that and build a base of aerobic fitness with a workout that combines walking with running. Below is an easy, get-up-to-speed plan for exercisers of two different fitness levels. In both the beginner and intermediate programs, take walk breaks as you need them. They'll help you avoid soreness, injury, and exhaustion, which means you'll be more likely to stick with the program.

WEEK 1	WORKOUT 1	WORKOUT 2	WORKOUT 3
Beginner	5-min walk 15-min run/walk (total: 20 min)	5-min walk 15-min run/walk (total: 20 min)	5-min walk 20-min run/walk 5-min walk (total: 30 min)
Intermediate (with walk breaks as needed)	30-min run	30-min run	30-min run

WEEKS 2 THROUGH 4	
Beginner	Increase running segments by 1 minute each week.
Intermediate	Add 5 minutes per week to this run, and try to eliminate walk breaks OR switch to the more intense interval workout found at the end of Chapter 5.

REAL GUYS—REAL RESULTS

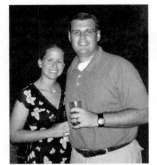

BEFORE:
278
POUNDS

AFTER:
180
POUNDS

"Losing weight helped me score my dream job."

VITALS: **Tyler Butts, 29, Frontenac, KS**
OCCUPATION: **Firefighter**
HEIGHT: **6'1"**
LESSON LEARNED: **You're much stronger than you think you are.**

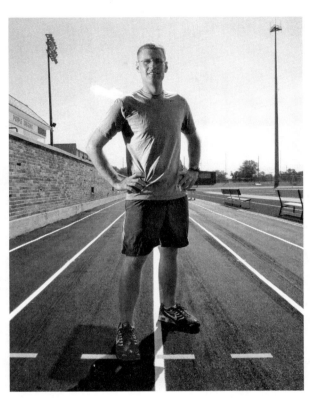

An athlete in high school, Tyler Butts stopped exercising after he graduated, and the flab started piling on—78 pounds in 5 years. "I just wasn't paying attention to how much I was eating," he says.

THE TURNING POINT

It happened on a scuba diving vacation. "I was struggling against the current just to get myself up into the boat," he says. "I realized I wasn't living the life I wanted." He also knew that he couldn't advance from volunteer to full-time firefighter unless he shaped up. He hired a personal trainer.

LIFE IN THE FIT LANE

Butts now visits the gym 5 days a week for an hour—30 minutes each of cardio and weight training. When the weather is nice, he runs outdoors. As a firefighter, he says, excuses are hard to come by. "You always have to be physically ready for the call, because the gear adds about 50 pounds to your frame." Butts eats a lot of whole grains, fruits, and vegetables, but his most effective dieting strategy is eating smaller portions.

THE REWARD

Besides landing his dream job in the fire department, Butts has become stronger both physically and mentally.

"When I started, I didn't know I would find this inner strength and it's really helped push me along," he says. "I've become more confident in every area of my life."

BUTTS'S BEST BELLY OFF! TIPS

●Get outside. Running to nowhere on a treadmill can sap your motivation. Running outside won't feel like a workout.

●Trick yourself into eating less. Portion your snacks into smaller bags so you're less likely to end up elbow deep in an economy-size bag of Lay's.

●Invest in yourself. Hiring a personal trainer makes it more difficult to skip workouts because someone is expecting you to show up and you've already paid. Too pricey? Get a discount by signing up a friend.

PART II

The Belly Off! Diet Workouts

5

BURN FAT WITH THE BODYWEIGHT 100 PROGRAM

An Easy 4-Week Plan. No Gym Required

THE BELLY OFF! CLUB grew from a humble beginning. Sometime during the early days of the summer of 2000, several *Men's Health* editors were playing our regular Wednesday lunchtime game of basketball at the court near our Pennsylvania offices. Shirts versus skins. I was one of the skins, along with writer Hugh O'Neill, editor Peter Moore, and fitness editor Lou Schuler. As we were comparing our scratches and bruises, Lou made an observation: We doughboys didn't look much like the guys on the cover of our magazine. In fact, we—the shirts included—were quite a bit softer than the ideal we put forward in our pages. So we thought: If we can tell our readers how to lose their bellies and build muscle, shouldn't we do these things ourselves?

Seven of us decided to give it a try. We hired a trainer—longtime *Men's Health* exercise consultant Mike Mejia—to design workouts for each of us, and we consulted nutritionists for customized diets. We took to the challenge like yellow-jacket wasps to orange soda. And the competitive atmosphere of our editorial offices only fanned the flames of our determination. We lifted weights at the company gym. Some of us took spinning classes. Others swam or biked. Everyone ran at lunchtime. And 6 weeks later, we were finished. We all had added muscle and trimmed our body-fat percentages; and those of us who needed to lost considerable weight. Some of us even found our abs. We all felt more like *Men's Health* editors in the end, so we chronicled our quest in a story, which ran in the October 2000 issue. In that article we also launched the *Men's Health* Belly Off! Club on our Web site, inviting readers to transform their bodies, too. Within a month, the club had more than 20,000 members sharing workouts, weight-loss and nutrition tips, and motivational support through our forums. Today, there are more than 300,000 men in the club. If you're not one of them, go to www.menshealth.com/bellyoff and sign up. It's free. There, you'll find more nutrition advice, useful tools, and workouts, including an advanced version of the Bodyweight 100 workout described on the following pages.

You are going to love the Bodyweight series of workouts. Why are we so sure? Because the workouts are designed to address everything you *don't* like about exercise.

Let's start with a few assumptions:

- ■ *You're a busy man.* You've got work and volunteer commitments, home duties, friends, and family with which to share your time. You don't have the luxury to spend hours in a gym like an underwear model. And that's fine. Join the club. But you *can* carve out 15 to 20 minutes three or four times a week if you put your mind to it, right?

- **You may not like going to a gym.** It may be too far away. Too expensive. Too full of grunting muscleheads and bad music. Maybe you feel a bit intimidated because of extra weight that you may be carrying around. No problem. We're not going there.

- **You don't have a fully equipped home gym.** In fact, you might not own anything but a pair of running shoes. That's fine, too. For the Belly Off! Bodyweight program, all you need is, well, you.

- **Barbells and fitness machines have their place.** And you may someday want to give them a try. But you don't have to use them to become leaner, fitter, and stronger.

- **You've tried exercise before and have always fallen off the wagon.** Don't beat yourself up. We've all done that. Polls show that 50 percent of people drop out of their exercise programs within 6 months. But we've got some tricks to keep you on this one.

- **Exercise is boring.** If you feel this way, it's probably because you're doing the same routine over and over, and you don't have a workout partner or some sort of motivational support system in place. Our plan is flexible and fun, it changes quickly to keep your interest, and it grows along with your muscles so there are always new ways to challenge your body.

Do these assumptions reflect some of your attitudes toward exercise? Then the fitness plan on the following pages is custom-made for you. Master it in the first 4 weeks. That's the crucial period. You'll start to see and feel results within just 5 days. And that motivation will carry you through until the Belly Off! Diet becomes a natural part of your new lifestyle.

FIT FACT

Just three 15-minute workouts a week can double a beginner's strength within a month, according to University of Kansas researchers.

THE BELLY OFF! DIET WORKOUT SCHEDULE

MONDAY	TUESDAY	WEDNESDAY	THURSDAY	FRIDAY	SATURDAY	SUNDAY
2-Minute Drill	2-Minute Drill	2-Minute Drill	2-Minute Drill	2-Minute Drill	2-Minute Drill	Rest
Bodyweight 100/200	Cardio Intervals	Bodyweight 100/200	Cardio Intervals	Bodyweight 100/200	Cardio Intervals	

FIT FACT

Pullups are terrific for building biceps. When West Point researchers measured muscle activity during the exercise, they found that pullups target the biceps just as much as the lats. And, think about it: when you do a pullup, you're using a weight that's much heavier than the weight you curl.

THE BODYWEIGHT 100 WORKOUTS

Pound for pound, gymnasts are perhaps the strongest athletes in the world. And most of them rarely, if ever, lift weights. You don't have to pump iron or use high-tech machines at the gym to build a strong and lean physique. Using the weight of your body alone is enough resistance to give yourself an exceptional workout. Bodyweight moves, after all, are the most natural of exercises and the least likely to cause injury.

Craig Ballantyne, a certified strength and conditioning specialist, longtime *Men's Health* contributor, and owner of Turbulencetraining.com, has developed the Bodyweight 100 to 500 program. (The full routine is found at www.menshealth.com/bellyoff.) The number refers to the total repetitions you end up doing in each circuit. For the first 2 weeks, we recommend you follow the Bodyweight 100 and 200 exercises. These moves will prepare your muscles for the next phase of the resistance workout, Weeks 3 and 4, and, later, when we introduce some weights into the routine for added variety.

WEEK 1:
THE BODYWEIGHT 100

The Bodyweight 100 is a terrific workout that takes very little time. Again, the number "100" refers to the total number of repetitions you will have done after completing the sixth exercise. Start the session by warming up your muscles with a few minutes of jumping jacks or running in place. Then do the following six calisthenics rapidly with no rest in between exercises. Rest for 2 minutes after you complete this circuit, then repeat the six exercises in the same order. If you feel you can push yourself through a third circuit, rest for another 2 minutes, then go for it.

EXERCISE	REPS
Prisoner Squats (page 82)	20 reps
Pushups (page 83)	20 reps
Jumps (page 84)	20 reps
Chinups (page 85)	20 reps
Forward Lunges (page 86)	20 reps
Close-Grip Pushups (page 87)	20 reps
REST	2 minutes

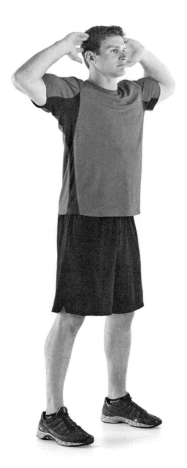

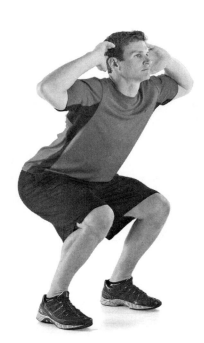

PRISONER SQUATS

Stand with your hands behind your ears, your chest out, your elbows back, and your feet hip-width apart. Sit back at your hips and bend your knees to lower your body as far as you can without losing the natural arch of your spine. Squeeze your gluteals and push yourself back to the starting position.

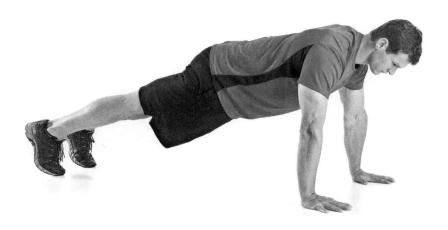

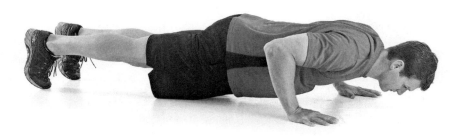

PUSHUPS

Get into the pushup position: back and legs straight, hands beneath your shoulders. Brace your abs and keep your body rigid. Now lower yourself until your chest nears the floor. Then push yourself up until your arms are extended.

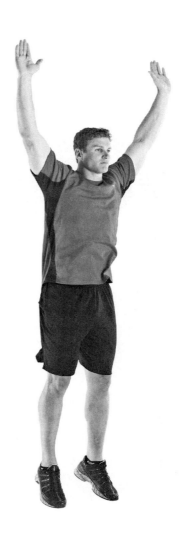
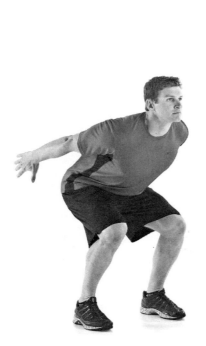

JUMPS

Stand with your feet slighty more than hip-width apart. Swing your arms back as you dip down at the hips and knees. Drive your arms forward and up as you jump explosively off the floor. Immediately dip down and repeat.

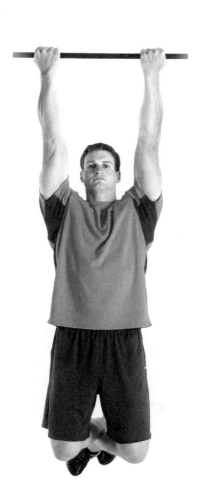
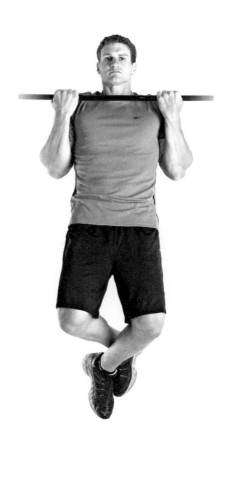

CHINUPS

Start from a full hang, hands shoulder-width apart, palms toward you. Pull your chin over the bar and then lower your body back down. Beginner's Tip: If you can't perform these at first, do "negative chinups." See "Conquer the Classic Pullup," on page 88 for a description.

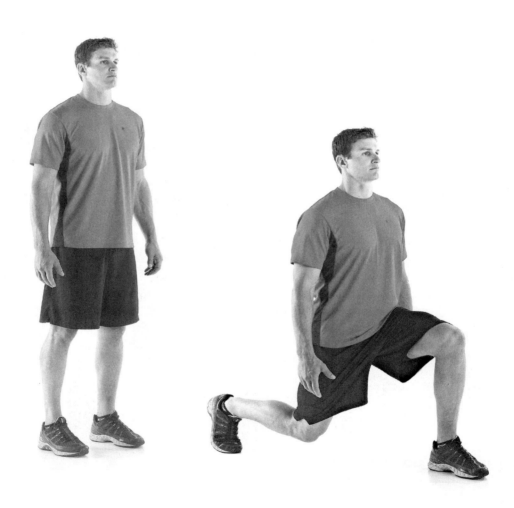

FORWARD LUNGES

From a standing position, take a large step forward with one leg. When your front thigh is parallel to the floor and keeping your back knee off the floor, hold for 1 second. Then return to the starting position and repeat with your other leg.

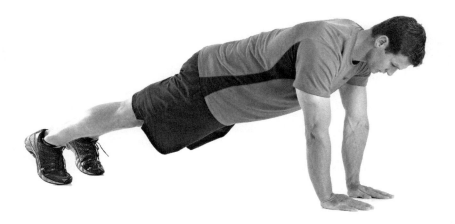

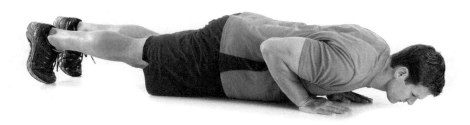

CLOSE-GRIP PUSHUPS

Assume the standard pushup position, but place your hands closer together, leaving about 4 inches of space between your thumbs. Keeping your elbows tucked in against your sides, lower yourself until your chest nears the floor, then push yourself up.

CONQUER THE CLASSIC PULLUP

"Negatives" Make This Tough Exercise Easier

Guys avoid pullups and chinups for mostly one reason: They're hard. And if you're carrying around even a little extra weight, you might find it nearly impossible to manage even one. That's a shame because you'd be missing out on the best way to work the biggest muscle group in your upper body: your latissimus dorsi, the set of fan-shaped muscles found along the sides of your body that spread across the width of your back. But here's a strategy for mastering the pullup that works.

TEST YOUR LIMIT

First, determine how many pullups you can do. Hang from a pullup bar using an overhand grip that's just beyond shoulder-width apart, your arms completely straight. Cross your feet behind you. Without moving your lower body, pull yourself as high as you can; your chin should rise above the bar. Pause momentarily, then lower your body until your arms are straight, and repeat. Record your total, then find the pullup routine below that corresponds to your best effort. Do that workout twice a week, resting at least 2 days between sessions. After 4 weeks, retest yourself. Depending on your score, either advance to the next workout or repeat the same routine for another 4 weeks.

0 TO 1 PULLUP

The fix: Heavy "negatives." Do only the lowering portion of the exercise. It will help you build strength for full pullups.

How to do it: First, a couple of definitions.

•**Chinup.** This is the same movement as a pullup, but you'll use a shoulder-width, underhand grip. Because your biceps are more involved, it's a little easier than the pullup.

•**Neutral-grip pullup.** Again, this is the same basic movement, but you'll grip the parallel bars of the pullup station so your palms are facing each other. This is harder than a chinup, but not as hard as a pullup.

Now follow the workout schedule below, using this method of performing negatives: Place a bench or chair under a pullup bar and use it to boost your body so your chin is above the bar. Then take the prescribed amount of time—either 5 to 6 seconds or 8 to 10 seconds—to lower your body. Once your arms are straight, jump back up to the top position and repeat. Rest for 60 seconds after each set.

WEEK	EXERCISE	SETS	REPS	TIME
1	Chinup	3	5–6	5–6 sec
2	Neutral-grip pullup	3	5–6	5–6 sec
3	Neutral-grip pullup	2	5–6	8–10 sec
4	Pullup	2	5–6	8–10 sec

2 TO 4 PULLUPS

The fix: Do more sets of fewer repetitions. The reason: The first one or two repetitions in a set are the "highest quality" ones, meaning that's when the most muscle fibers fire. By doing several sets of 1 or 2 repetitions, you'll activate more total fibers and better develop the communication pathways between your brain and muscle—increasing strength quickly.

How to do it: Take the number of pullups you can complete and divide it by 2. That's how many repetitions you'll do in each set. (If your best effort is three, round down to one.) Follow the workout routine below, doing the number of sets indicated and resting for the prescribed amount of time after each. Note that after 2 weeks, you'll increase the repetitions you do in each set.

WEEK	SETS	REPS	REST
1	8	50% of best effort	90 sec
2	8	50% of best effort	90 sec
3	8	Best effort	90 sec
4	8	Best effort	90 sec

5 TO 7 PULLUPS

The fix: To improve muscular endurance, focus on doing more total repetitions than normal—regardless of the number of sets it takes. For instance, instead of doing 3 sets of 6 repetitions, for a total of 18, you'll shoot for 30 repetitions—even if that means you have to drop down to sets of 3, 2, or 1. This will rapidly improve your muscular endurance.

How to do it: Perform as many pullups as you can, then rest for 60 seconds. Repeat as many times as needed to do 30 repetitions. Each workout, try to reach your goal in fewer sets.

WEEK 2:
THE BODYWEIGHT 200

This week, we're adding five new bodyweight exercises to the workout and increasing the total number of repetitions to 200. Also, we're throwing a new toy into the mix—a stability ball, also known as a Swiss ball.

Stability balls should really be called "instability balls," because that's the secret to how they work. Supporting yourself with the ball creates instability, which forces you to use more muscles to help you balance while exercising on it, says Rafael Escamilla, PhD, a professor of physical therapy at California State University, Sacramento. That equals better and faster results. In a recent study, Escamilla and colleagues hooked electrodes to the torsos of 18 people to measure muscle stimulation while some of them exercised on a stability ball and others exercised without the ball. The researchers found that the stability ball crunches recruited twice the number of muscle fibers as traditional crunches or yoga/Pilates-inspired workouts. Another study in New Zealand found that pushups using a stability ball trained arms 30 percent harder than regular pushups did. "The Swiss ball forces your triceps to stabilize your elbow and shoulder joints, which results in the recruitment of more muscle fibers," according to lead investigator, Paul Marshal, MS.

ROLL MODEL
How to Buy a Stability Ball

Most men between 5'8" and 6'1" will need a 25.5-inch (or 65-cm) stability ball. You can buy one at sporting goods stores or online for around $30 with a pump. We like the Resist-A-Ball (power-systems.com) and Gymnic Plus (performbetter.com) because they're made with burst-resistant latex-free vinyl and will deflate slowly if punctured.

After warming up, do the Bodyweight 200. Note the increase in repetitions. If you are spent after the 200 reps, stop. If you can bang out another circuit after a 5-minute rest, go for it.

EXERCISE	REPS
Prisoner Squats (page 82)	30 reps
Pushups (page 83)	30 reps
Jumps (page 84)	10 reps
Stability Ball Leg Curls (page 92)	10 reps
Stability Ball Jackknifes (page 93)	10 reps
Stepups (page 94)	20 reps
Pullups (page 95)	5 reps
Forward Lunges (page 86)	30 reps
Close-Grip Pushups (page 87)	20 reps
Inverted Rows (page 101)	15 reps
Prisoner Squats (page 82)	15 reps
Chinups (page 85)	5 reps
REST	5 minutes

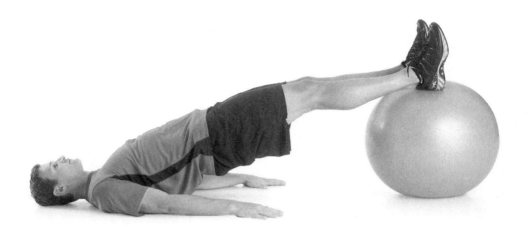

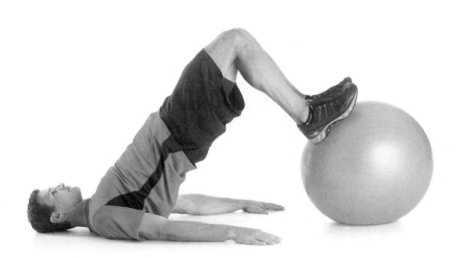

STABILITY BALL LEG CURLS

Lie on the floor with your calves on a stability ball and your arms at your sides. Squeeze your gluteals to raise your hips off the floor so your body is in a straight line from your shoulders to your ankles. Pause for a second, then bend your legs to roll the ball toward your butt. Straighten your legs to roll the ball back out away from you, then lower your body to the floor.

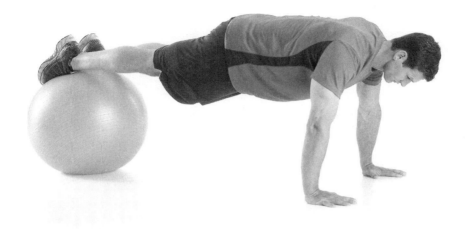

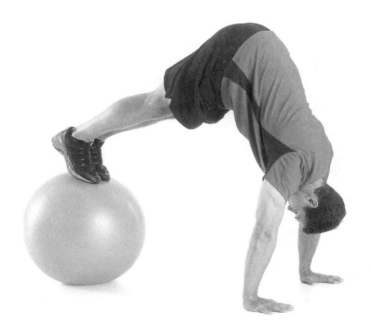

STABILITY BALL JACKKNIFES

Get into a pushup position with the tops of your feet resting on a stability ball, your body forming a straight line from toes to shoulders. Keep your back straight as you contract your abs and roll the ball toward you.

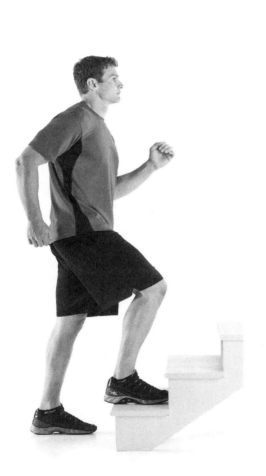
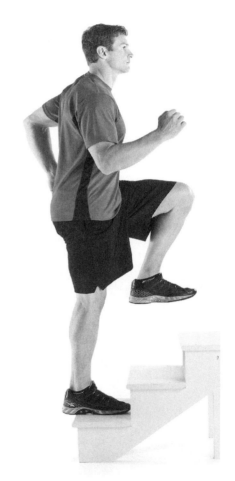

STEPUPS

Place one foot on a step or bench and push down through your heel to lift your other leg up. Return to the starting position and finish all reps with one leg before switching legs and repeating the exercise.

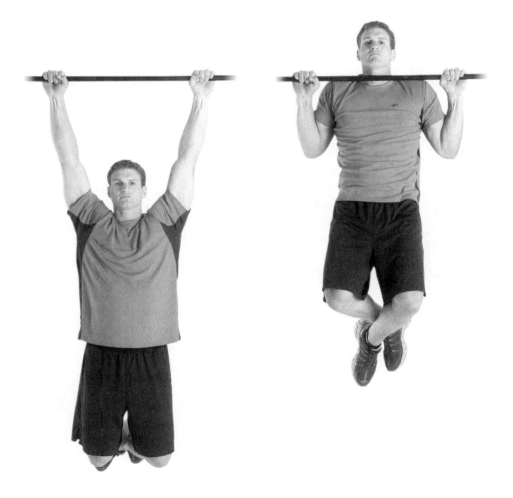

PULLUPS

Start from a full hang, hands shoulder-width apart, palms facing
away from you. Pull your chin over the bar and then lower your body
back down.

WEEK 3:
THE BODYWEIGHT 200, 2X

Complete the Bodyweight 200 twice, with 5 minutes of rest between circuits. Too hard? Then do another week of the Bodyweight 200. Too easy? Then try the Bodyweight 200, plus the Bodyweight 100 exercises, with no rest between circuits. It's your call.

EXERCISE	REPS
Prisoner Squats (page 82)	30 reps
Pushups (page 83)	30 reps
Jumps (page 84)	10 reps
Stability Ball Leg Curls (page 92)	10 reps
Stability Ball Jackknifes (page 93)	10 reps
Stepups (page 94)	20 reps
Pullups (page 95)	5 reps
Forward Lunges (page 86)	30 reps
Close-grip Pushups (page 87)	20 reps
Inverted Rows (page 101)	15 reps
Prisoner Squats (page 82)	15 reps
Chinups (page 85)	5 reps
REST	5 minutes

WEEKS 4 TO 6: BODYWEIGHT SUPERSETS

You can keep doing these Bodyweight workouts for months, mixing up the exercises to suit your mood and keep challenging your muscles. Or you can follow the specific workouts through to the Bodyweight 500 on the Belly Off! Club Web site.

But I suggest we change things up for the next 2 weeks by doing Bodyweight Supersets. A superset is nothing more than a workout technique that pairs two different exercises back-to-back without a rest. Supersets are designed to save time and burn fat by multitasking your muscles. For example, you might work your chest and back in one superset and your legs and shoulders in another. By stressing your muscles in a short time period, you increase the rate at which your body breaks down and rebuilds protein, and this uptick in your metabolism can last for hours after your workout.

To get the most out of supersets, use compound and combination moves—exercises that work multiple muscle groups across multiple joints rather than focusing on just one muscle. By pairing noncompeting muscle groups such as your shoulders and your legs as suggested in the following workouts, you'll be able to push yourself even harder. Your back and deltoids will be able to rest while your hams, gluteals, and calves work during the leg exercises. You'll be able to jump into your next set that much quicker, saving time. Here are two different superset workouts. Do Workout A on Monday and B on Wednesday, then go back to Workout A on Friday and so on, in alternating fashion.

SUPERSHOT
Forge a
Viselike Grip

Strengthening your grip will help you do pullups by allowing you to transfer more force from your arms to the bar and ensure that your forearms won't give out before your back does. Do the farmer's walk: Grab a heavy dumbbell in each hand, let your arms hang naturally at your sides, and walk across the room. Use the heaviest pair of dumbbells that allows you to walk for 60 seconds. Do 3 or 4 sets, resting 60 seconds after each rep.

SUPERSET WORKOUT A

Superset 1	
Shoulder Press Pushup (page 99)	10 reps
Stepup (page 99)	12 reps per leg
REST	1 minute
Shoulder Press Pushup	10 reps
Stepup	12 reps per leg
REST	1 minute
Shoulder Press Pushup	10 reps
Stepup	12 reps per leg
REST	5 minutes
Superset 2	
Single-Leg Good Morning (page 100)	8 reps per leg
Swiss Ball Mountain Climber (page 100)	20 reps
REST	1 minute
Single-Leg Good Morning	8 reps per leg
Swiss Ball Mountain Climber	20 reps
REST	1 minute
Single-Leg Good Morning	8 reps per leg
Swiss Ball Mountain Climber	20 reps
REST	5 minutes
Superset 3	
Inverted Row (page 101)	12 reps
Wide-Grip Pushup (page 101)	20 reps
REST	1 minute
Inverted Row	12 reps
Wide-Grip Pushup	20 reps
REST	1 minute
Inverted Row	12 reps
Wide-Grip Pushup	20 reps
REST	5 minutes

SUPERSET WORKOUT █A█

Perform these two exercises back-to-back, no rest in between. Rest 1 minute before repeating Superset 1 twice more. Then rest 5 minutes and move to Superset 2.

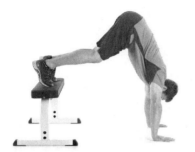 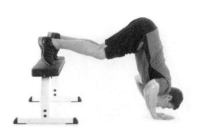

Shoulder Press Pushup (10 reps)

Place your feet on a bench, step, or chair and your hands on the floor slightly wider than shoulder width. Pike your hips in the air, so that your body forms an upside-down V and your upper body is as vertical as can be. Slowly lower your head to the floor. Pause, and push with your shoulders and triceps back to the starting position.

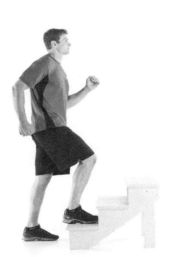 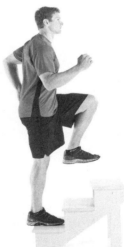

Stepup (12 reps per leg)

Place one foot on the step and push down through your heel to lift your other leg up. Return to the starting position and finish all the repetitions with one leg before repeating the exercise with your other leg. To make the exercise more difficult, use a bench or place your foot on the second step.

SUPERSET WORKOUT **A**

Perform these two exercises back-to-back, no rest in between. Rest 1 minute before repeating the superset two more times. Rest 5 minutes before moving to Superset 3.

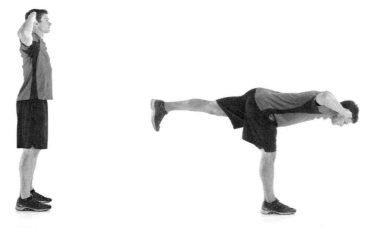

Single-Leg Good Morning (8 reps per leg)

Stand with your feet slightly more than shoulder-width apart and your hands behind your head so that your fingertips brush your ears. Raise one foot and extend it behind you. Contract your glutes, brace your abs, and keep your spine naturally arched. Focus on maintaining your balance, and lower yourself until your torso is parallel to the floor. Initiate the movement by pushing your hips back. Push back up to the starting position.

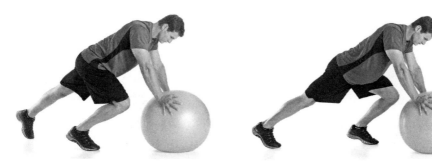

Swiss Ball Mountain Climber (20 reps)

Assume the pushup position, but place your hands on the sides of a stability ball, fingers pointing forward. Brace your abs and straighten your legs behind you. This is the starting position. Lift one foot off the floor and bring your knee toward your chest. Straighten your leg back out, move your other knee to your chest, and return that leg to the starting position. Keep alternating legs.

SUPERSET WORKOUT ◼A◼

Perform these two exercises back-to-back, no rest in between. Rest 1 minute before repeating the superset two more times.

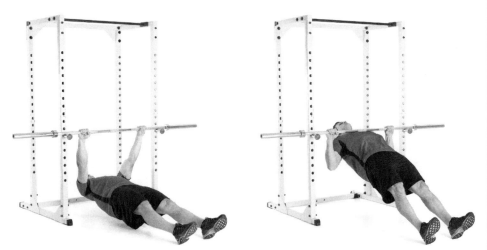

Inverted Row (12 reps)
Set your chinup bar in a doorway at about 3 feet from the floor or use a barbell and rack as shown. Lie faceup underneath the bar with your heels on the floor and grab the bar with your hands a little more than shoulder-width apart. Keeping your body in a straight line, pull your chest to the bar using your back muscles. Slowly lower yourself until your arms are straight.

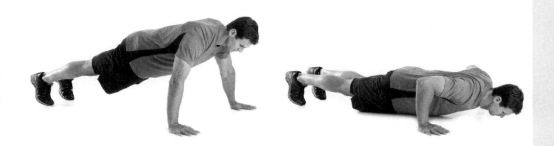

Wide-Grip Pushup (20 reps)
Do this as you would a standard pushup, but place your hands wider apart.

SUPERSET 3

SUPERSET WORKOUT B

Superset 1	
Prisoner Squats (page 103)	15 reps
Walking Offset Pushups (page 103)	8 reps per side
REST	1 minute
Prisoner Squats	15 reps
Walking Offset Pushups	8 reps per side
REST	1 minute
Prisoner Squats	15 reps
Walking Offset Pushups	8 reps per side
REST	5 minutes
Superset 2	
Split Squats with Front Foot Elevated (page 104)	12 reps per side
Inverted Rows (page 104)	12 reps
REST	1 minute
Split Squats with Front Foot Elevated	12 reps per side
Inverted Rows	12 reps
REST	1 minute
Split Squats with Front Foot Elevated	12 reps per side
Inverted Rows	12 reps
REST	5 minutes
Superset 3	
Stability Ball Jackknife Rotations (page 105)	6 reps per side
Stability Ball Leg Curls (page 105)	12 reps
REST	1 minute
Stability Ball Jackknife Rotations	6 reps per side
Stability Ball Leg Curls	12 reps
REST	1 minute
Stability Ball Jackknife Rotations	6 reps per side
Stability Ball Leg Curls	12 reps
REST	5 minutes
Superset 4	
Spiderman Pushups (page 106)	8 reps per side
Single-Leg Hip Extensions (page 106)	15 reps per side
REST	1 minute
Spiderman Pushups	8 reps per side
Single-Leg Hip Extension	15 reps per side
REST	1 minute
Spiderman Pushups	8 reps per side
Single-Leg Hip Extensions	15 reps per side
REST	5 minutes

SUPERSET WORKOUT **B**

Perform these two exercises back-to-back, no rest in between. Rest 1 minute before repeating the superset two more times, then move on to Superset 2.

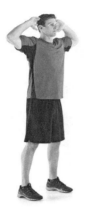
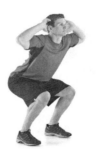

SUPERSET 1

Prisoner Squat (15 reps)
Stand with your hands behind your head so that your fingertips brush your ears, your chest out, and your elbows back. Sit back at your hips and bend your knees to lower your body as far as you can without losing the natural arch of your spine. Squeeze your gluteals and push yourself back to the starting position.

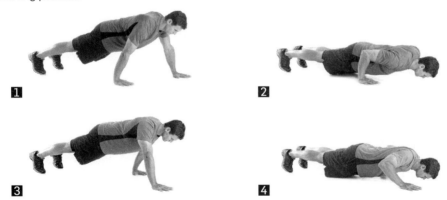

Walking Offset Pushup (8 reps per side)
(1) Place your hands on the floor slightly wider than shoulder-width apart, but place your left hand about 6 inches in front of your left shoulder and your right hand about 6 inches behind your right shoulder. (2) Using this staggered stance, slowly lower yourself until your chest is an inch off the ground. Push through your chest, shoulders, and triceps to return to the starting position. Keep your body in a straight line at all times. Do 2 reps for one side then (3) switch hand positions—that is, move your left hand behind your left shoulder and your right hand in front of your right shoulder—by "walking" one step forward. (4) Do 2 reps then "walk" forward again, repeating until you've completed 8 reps per side.

SUPERSET WORKOUT B

Perform these two exercises back-to-back, no rest in between. Rest 1 minute before repeating the superset two more times, then move on to Superset 3.

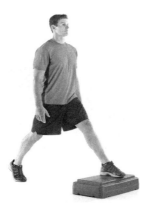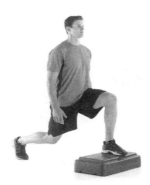

Split Squat with Front Foot Elevated (12 reps per side)
Stand with one foot 2 to 3 feet in front of the other, each in line with its corresponding buttock. Place the front foot on a 6-inch riser or step. Keep your upper body erect as you descend until the top of your front thigh is parallel to the ground. Pause, then press back up to the starting position.

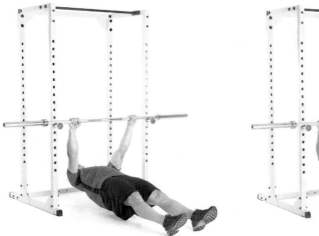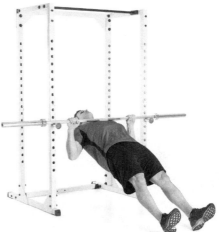

Inverted Row (12 reps)
Lie faceup underneath a bar with your heels on the floor and grab the bar with your hands a little more than shoulder-width apart. Keeping your body in a straight line, pull your chest to the bar using your back muscles. Slowly lower yourself until your arms are straight.

SUPERSET WORKOUT **B**

Perform these two exercises back-to-back, no rest in between. Rest 1 minute before repeating the superset two more times, then move on to Superset 4.

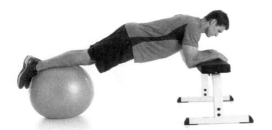
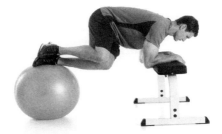

Stability Ball Jackknife Rotation (6 reps per side)
Brace your abs. Put your forearms on the bench and rest your shins on the stability ball. With your arms straight and your back flat, your body should form a straight line from your shoulders to your ankles. Keeping your back straight, roll the ball to your chest and bring your knees to one side of your body by contracting your abs and pulling the ball forward. Pause and then return the ball to the starting position by rolling it backward. Alternate sides.

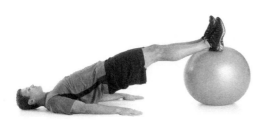
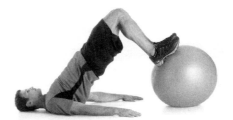

Stability Ball Leg Curl (12 reps)
Lie on the floor with your heels on a stability ball and your arms at your sides. Squeeze your glutes to raise your hips off of the floor so your body is in a straight line from your shoulders to your ankles. Pause for a second, then bend your legs to roll the ball toward your butt. Straighten your legs to roll the ball back out away from you, then lower your body to the floor.

SUPERSET 3

SUPERSET WORKOUT B

Perform these two exercises back-to-back, no rest in between. Rest 1 minute before repeating the superset two more times.

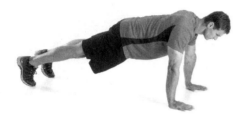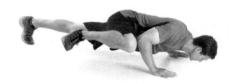

Spiderman Pushup (8 reps per side)

Assume the classic pushup position. Keeping your abs braced and your body in a straight line, slowly bend your elbows until your chest is a few inches from the floor. As you go down, bring your right knee to your right elbow. Straighten your leg back as you use your chest, shoulders, and triceps to push yourself back to the starting position. Alternate legs, doing 8 reps per side.

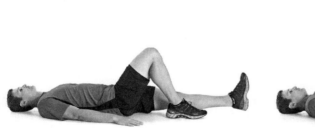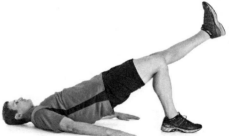

Single-Leg Hip Extension (15 reps per side)

Lie on your back with your knees bent and feet flat on the floor. Brace your abs while you take your left leg, straighten it, lift it off the floor, and point it straight ahead. Raise your hips so your body forms a straight line from your shoulders to your knees. Slowly lower your hips until they are an inch above the ground. Perform all reps for the left leg and then repeat the exercise with your right leg extended.

REAL GUYS—REAL RESULTS

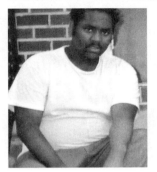

BEFORE:
234
POUNDS

AFTER:
150
POUNDS

"Girls pull me onto the dance floor."

VITALS: **Dennis McIver, 24, Baltimore, MD**
OCCUPATION: **Graduate student**
HEIGHT: **5'7"**
LESSON LEARNED: **Use life accomplishments to gain the confidence to stick to a weight-loss plan.**

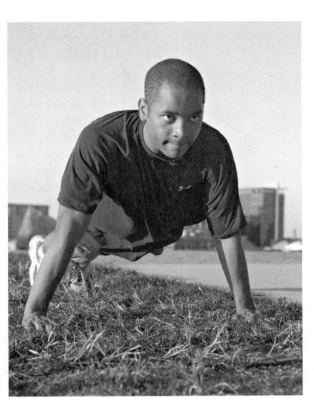

As a graduate assistant after college, McIver had unlimited access to the dining-hall buffet. "We had a burger station, a pizza station, and a dessert station," McIver says. "If I had trouble deciding, I would just say, 'It's free, so I'm having all three.'" With all-consuming schoolwork and no exercise, his belly ballooned.

THE TURNING POINT

McIver looked in the mirror and suddenly saw a fat man staring back. The needle on the scale spun to 234. "That's when it hit me." McIver decided to bring his physique up to the level of his intellectual accomplishments. "Having done well in school and gotten to the point in my life where I was supporting myself, I wanted to take it to the next level."

LIFE IN THE FIT LANE

McIver traded in the buffet-line burgers for turkey sandwiches, and pizza for chicken Caesar salad. He started cooking for himself so he had full control of what he ate. He began biking. "Cardio really helped me reinforce my diet," McIver says. "If I'm exercising four times a week and losing weight, why ruin it by eating poorly?" When he dropped to 140 pounds, he started lifting weights to pack on muscle.

THE REWARD

Bouncers at bars thought he was using a fake ID and refused to let him in. Longtime friends didn't recognize him. He's more confident meeting people. "It's thrilling to have girls pull me out onto the dance floor for a change," he says. McIver, however, is proudest of convincing his mom to lose weight. "With all she's done for me, it's the least I can do in return."

McIVER'S BEST BELLY OFF! TIPS

●Start out slow to avoid burning out. Set small goals until you are up and running.

●Cook your own meals. Preparing your own food gives you the ultimate control over your diet.

●Use workouts as reminders. It's less tempting to cheat with your diet when you feel like you're sabotaging the effort you put into that workout.

THE BELLY OFF! DIET INTERVAL WORKOUTS

While the Bodyweight 100 series and the Superset workouts will get your heart pumping, we recommend adding interval training on the days in between your strength workouts. As we said earlier, intervals are short bursts of high-intensity work interspersed with recovery periods of easier effort. You can do intervals with just about any type of exercise—cycling, running, rowing, swimming, jumping rope, or exercising on an elliptical trainer or a stairclimber.

You may have heard that long, slow runs are great for burning calories. Well, actually, recent studies show exercising at a higher intensity for a short period of time burns many more calories than long aerobic sessions do. Sprints fry more fat than distance running does—and a lot quicker. Canadian researchers found that high-intensity intervals were nine times more effective than endurance training at eliminating body fat. What's more, the higher the intensity of your interval workout, the longer your body will continue to burn fat and calories *after* you are finished exercising. This is known as afterburn, and it's the same benefit you get from rigorous weight-lifting. The bottom line is this: If you want to incinerate fat, you have to increase the intensity of your workouts.

On the next page are some examples of simple running interval workouts. You should perform them on the days in between your strength workouts or, if you feel ambitious, right after a resistance workout. Before each workout, warm up for 5 minutes by exercising at an easy pace (about 30 percent of your full effort). After you're finished, cool down for 5 minutes in the same manner.

INTERVAL WORKOUT 1	INTERVAL WORKOUT 2	INTERVAL WORKOUT 3
—Run for 30 seconds at 90 percent of your best effort.	—Run for 60 seconds at 80 percent of your best effort.	—Run for 90 seconds at 70 percent of your best effort.
—Slow down to about 30 percent of your best effort for 90 seconds.	—Slow down to about 30 percent of your best effort for 60 seconds.	—Slow down to about 30 percent of your best effort for 180 seconds.
—Repeat six to eight times.	—Repeat four to six times.	—Repeat two to four times.

Running over undulating hills or even a long, steady climb can create a natural interval workout. Run as fast as you can for as long as you can up the hill, then slow jog or walk until you've caught your breath, and repeat.

I find it easier (and safer) to do my intervals on a stationary cycle, spinning bike, or by hooking my road bike up to a magnetic resistance trainer. Here's my road bike workout: After a warmup, I'll go all out for 30 seconds, then recover for 30 seconds. I'll do 10 cycles of that sequence, then pedal hard for 60 seconds followed by 60 seconds of recovery pedaling for 5 sets. Finally, I'll pedal for another 5 minutes, this time changing gears to increase or decrease resistance at 15- to 30-second intervals.

THE WORLD'S BEST TOTAL-BODY STRETCH

Here's the Only Flexibility Routine You'll Ever Have to Do—
and It Takes Just 2 Minutes!

While she was stretching my hamstrings, a personal trainer once told me that I was the most inflexible man she had ever met. "Funny," I said, "my wife tells me that all the time."

But I'm not alone. Few guys are what you'd call limber. Because few guys like to stretch. Because it hurts. Our legs are naturally more muscular than women's legs, which makes our hamstrings tight. Running exacerbates the problem. And stress doesn't help our flexibility. We tend to carry stress around in the form of tense shoulder, back, and neck muscles. All this puts us at risk for pulled muscles, overuse injuries, and tension pain. So, do yourself a favor and learn to like stretching, or at least learn to endure it until you loosen up and it becomes more fun.

This five-part stretching routine is based on some classic, yet simple, yoga moves, with a slight twist. It's terrific because it will help you loosen up your chest, abs, hamstrings, back, calves, and arms—nearly every major muscle group. The bird-dog stretch is particularly useful because it strengthens the lower back, one of the most vulnerable spots on a man's body. That makes it ideal for men who spend an inordinate amount of time sitting in a desk chair. Visit www.menshealth.com/bellyoff to watch a video of these stretches.

Do the following routine after every workout. But don't limit it just to workouts. You can do it any time of day when you're feeling tight from stress. The multitasker in me likes cranking out a set while watching TV.

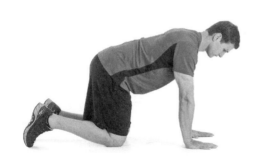

1 Get down on all fours with your hands and feet about shoulder-width apart, palms resting flat on the floor, your back straight and head in alignment with your back; you are facing the floor.

2 Do the bird-dog. Lift your right leg out straight behind you while simultaneously lifting your left arm straight out in front of you. Hold for a second or two, then lift your left leg out behind you and your right arm out in front. Continue alternating until you've completed 10 repetitions.

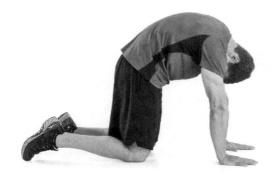

3 Return to position 1. Now slowly drop your head and round your back upward as shown in the photo. Keep your hands and knees on the ground throughout the stretch. Hold it for 30 seconds.

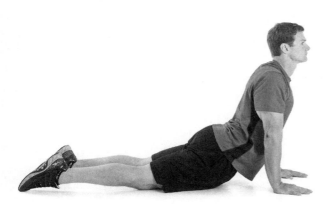

4 Next raise your head up while lowering your hips toward the ground and arching your back. Your head should point toward the ceiling. Feel the stretch? Contract your shoulder blades to open up your chest. Hold for 30 seconds.

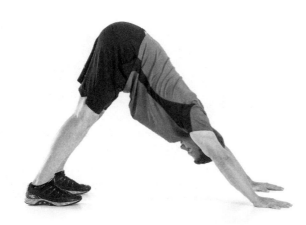

5 Finally, slowly lift your butt, straightening your legs while pointing the top of your head to the floor. Your body should form an upside-down V. Your feet should be flat on the floor. Try to keep your heels down. You'll feel the stretch in your hamstrings and back. Hold for 30 seconds.

6

PICK UP
A FEW POUNDS
How Lifting Dumbbells Can Build
More Muscle and Fry More Fat

D **ID I MENTION** that after about age 30, men tend to lose some muscle mass with each passing year? Unfair, isn't it? It means my body will probably never be as Speedo-friendly as it was on my honeymoon. (Maybe that's a good thing.) More important, it means that with less muscle, my metabolism is slower and it will be easier for fat to accumulate, especially around my middle. Hey, same goes for you, if you're over 30. And you know how dangerous abdominal fat can be.

Fortunately, the bodyweight resistance exercises you've been doing can counteract that phenomenon. Now we're going to make your strength workouts even more effective by adding weights to the program. There's still no reason to join a gym. You can continue to work out at home. But you do need to purchase a pair or two of dumbbells, say, a set of 20- to 30-pounders—

SUPERSHOT
Forced March

Park a block away from where you need to go. The extra walking can burn an additional 30 calories. Do this every day and you could lose 3 pounds of fat in a year.

depending on your level of strength—and a set of 35- to 45-pounders. Round out your equipment with a stability ball and a weight bench, and that's all you need to work your entire body at home.

As you learned earlier, how much your metabolism stays fired up after your workout is directly related to the amount of muscle tissue you engage. So, our new dumbbell workout targets the largest muscle groups in the body—the chest, back, shoulders, and legs. A University of Wisconsin study found that when men performed a full-body workout involving just three big-muscle exercises—the bench press, power clean, and squat—their metabolisms were elevated for 39 hours afterward! In addition, researchers discovered that these lifters also burned a greater percentage of their calories from fat during this time, compared with guys who didn't do a total-body, big-muscle workout. Many of the exercises in this program go one step further: They combine two lifts into one exercise to work multiple large muscle groups to deliver an even better metabolism charge while saving you workout time.

Here are some more reasons to add weights to your workout—and to make them dumbbells:

- Weights push your muscles harder. Once your body gets used to doing the exercises in the Bodyweight program, your muscles will stop growing. Seasoned weight lifters call this phenomenon *plateauing*. You reach a level at which your exercise isn't as effective. But by adding weights to your training, your muscles will stay challenged and continue to grow.

- Weight training strengthens your bones and your heart. Studies have shown that lifting weights can reduce your blood pressure, make your heart pump blood more efficiently, and reduce the amount of artery-clogging choles-terol. Other studies indicate that the act of stressing your skeleton with weights can even make your bones less prone to fracture.

IT WORKS FOR ME

"Pick a goal that will reward you with an experience, like training for a 10-K."

—Thomas Derr,
Madison, WI,
who lost 70 pounds

- Dumbbells build bigger muscles. Because dumbbells allow a greater range of motion, you can work out in three dimensions rather than the static up-and-down or side-to-side motions to which barbells and machines limit you. This helps you engage more muscle fibers with each rep. Personally, I prefer dumbbells because they are easier on my wrists. Barbells lock my wrists into a position that presses on nerves and causes me carpal-tunnel-like pain. But dumbbells let me adjust my wrists to help take the pressure off during certain lifts.

- Free weights force your body to do a balancing act. Unlike exercise machines that do the balancing for you, when you lift barbells and dumbbells, your body must constantly make minor adjustments so you don't fall over or drop the weights. This engages tiny muscle fibers that wouldn't normally be stressed during machine-based workouts. Bottom line: more muscle engaged, more calories burned, and more muscle grown.

FAT FACT

$2^1/_2$

Hours you would have to spend shoveling snow in order to burn off the 1,396 calories in a Denny's Extreme Grand Slam breakfast (2 eggs, bacon, sausage, pancakes, and hash browns) and large orange juice

IRON WORKS
The Original Hulk Says the Genius of Dumbbells Is Their Simplicity

Several years ago I asked Lou Ferrigno about his favorite piece of workout equipment. "The dumbbell," he said without hesitation.

Ferrigno told me that his Uncle Joe, a plumber, had given him his first set. "I was very young, and they changed my life," said the former Mr. Universe (1973, 1974), who played the Incredible Hulk in the TV series of the same name from 1977 to 1981. "I was a shy boy. I had 80 percent hearing loss. But those dumbbells helped me overcome my handicap and my shyness."

The dumbbell is perfectly designed. Small in size, with a handle balanced by equal weights at each end, it lets you put your muscles through a greater range of motion than any other weight-lifting tool does. With a pair of dumbbells, you can exercise almost every muscle in your body.

"When I was making the movie *Hercules*, there was no gym near our location, so I bought some dumbbells," recalled Ferrigno. "That was all I needed. No single piece of exercise equipment has ever surpassed the usefulness of the simple dumbbell."

THE BELLY OFF! DIET DUMBBELL WORKOUTS

Before you get started, there's a law of muscle physics to learn that'll help you get quicker results from your lifting. It's the law of "elastic energy." When you lower the weight during any exercise, you build up elastic energy in your muscles. Just like in a coiled spring, that elasticity allows you to bounce back to the starting position, reducing the work your muscles have to do. I call it unconscious cheating. But if you eliminate this cheating bounce, you'll force your body to recruit more muscle fibers to get you moving again. So pause for about 3 seconds in the down position of an exercise. That's the amount of time it takes to discharge all the elastic energy of a muscle.

There's another benefit to this strategy: Lowering a weight with control will force your muscles to work harder, stimulating more growth and burning more calories. According to a study in the *Journal of Strength and Conditioning Research*, men can handle 40 percent more weight on the eccentric, or lowering, portion of a bench press than on the press itself. So you can actually increase size and strength by targeting the down phase of a lift. Keep these points in mind as you do the following dumbbell exercises.

Alternate Workouts A and B, over 3 lifting days each week. Do 2 sets of 8 to 12 repetitions each. That'll take you 15 to 20 minutes.

SUPERSHOT
Go Nowhere Faster

Decision time at the gym: rowing machine or stationary cycle? Choose rowing. Researchers measuring the amount of fat used for fuel while men exercised on either a rowing machine or stationary cycle found that participants burned 40 percent more fat while rowing. Why? They believe it's because rowing engages more muscle, both your upper and lower body, than cycling, which focuses on the legs only.

DUMBBELL WORKOUT A

Bulgarian Split Squat	8-12 reps per leg
Dumbbell Stepup	8-12 reps per leg
Dumbbell Bench Press	8-12 reps
Seated Dumbbell Shoulder Press	8-12 reps
Biceps Curl	8-12 reps
Dumbbell Single-Arm Row	8-12 reps per arm
Crunch	1 set to failure

WORKOUT **A**

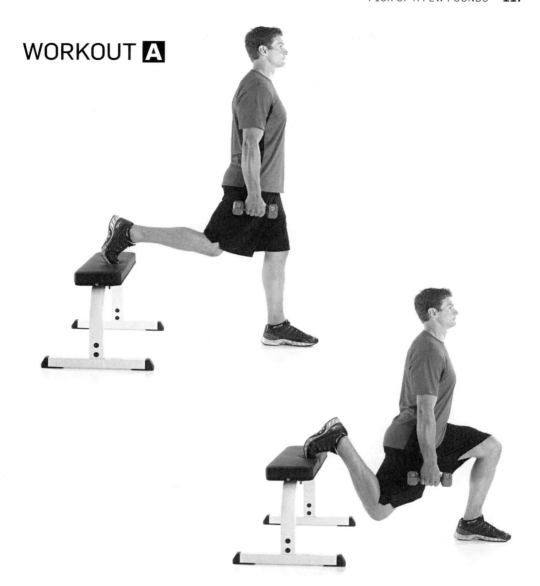

BULGARIAN SPLIT SQUAT

Grab a pair of dumbbells and stand with your back 2 to 3 feet from a bench. Place your right foot behind you on the bench so that your foot rests on it. Hold the dumbbells at arm's length at your sides. Keeping your torso upright, lower your body until your left knee is bent 90 degrees and your right knee nearly touches the floor. Pause, then push yourself back to the starting position as quickly as you can. Do 8 to 12 repetitions, then place your left foot on the bench and repeat the exercise this time with your left foot behind you on the bench.

WORKOUT **A**

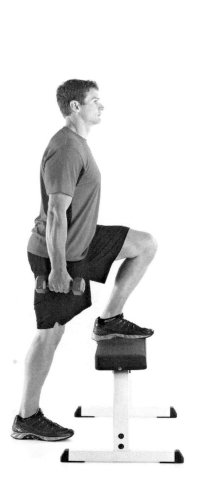

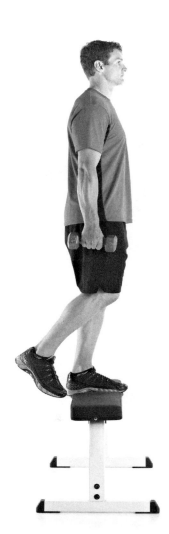

DUMBBELL STEPUP

Grab a pair of dumbbells and hold them at arm's length at your sides. Stand in front of a bench or a sturdy chair, and place your left foot on it. Press your left heel into the bench and push your body up until your left leg is straight and you're standing on one leg on the bench. Lower your body until your right foot touches the floor. That's 1 repetition. Do 8 to 12 reps with your left leg, then repeat the exercise with your right leg.

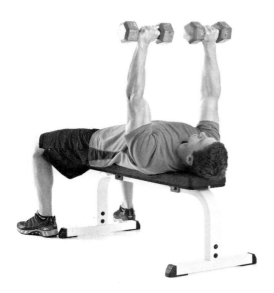

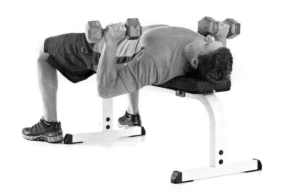

DUMBBELL BENCH PRESS

Lie on a flat bench holding a pair of dumbbells above your chest, with your back in a normal arch. Lower the dumbbells toward the sides of your chest (stop when your elbows are at torso level or just a little lower), pause, then push them back up to the starting position.

WORKOUT **A**

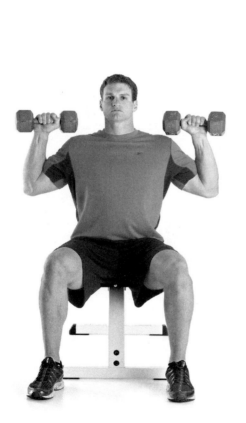
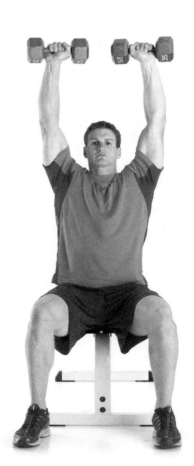

SEATED DUMBBELL SHOULDER PRESS

Sit on an exercise bench holding a pair of dumbbells. Lift the dumbbells up just above your shoulders and, with your feet flat on the floor, press the weights up until your arms are straight. Pause, lower, and repeat. You can also do this exercise with a neutral grip to ease strain on your shoulder joints.

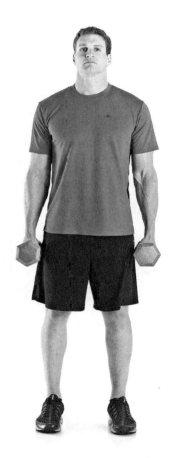
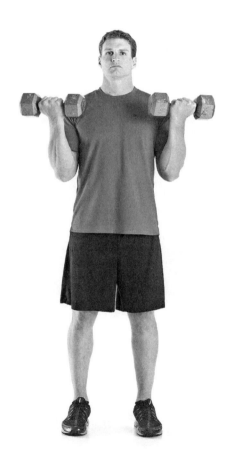

BICEPS CURL

Stand holding a pair of dumbbells at your sides. Keeping your upper arms perfectly still, curl the weights up with an underhand grip in front of your shoulders. Pause, lower, and repeat.

WORKOUT A

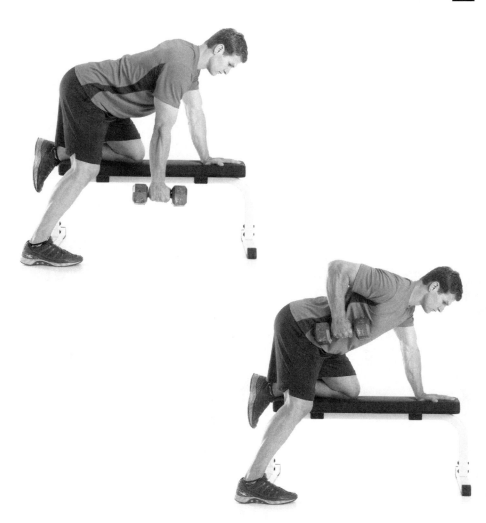

DUMBBELL SINGLE-ARM ROW

Grab a dumbbell in your right hand and place your left hand and left knee on a flat bench. Keep your back flat and your upper body parallel to the floor. Let your right arm hang straight down from your shoulder with your palm facing your torso. Raise your right upper arm up until it's just past parallel to the floor, with your elbow above the level of your torso. Pause, lower, and repeat. Do 8 to 12 reps, then repeat the exercise using your left hand holding the dumbbell and your right hand and knee on the bench.

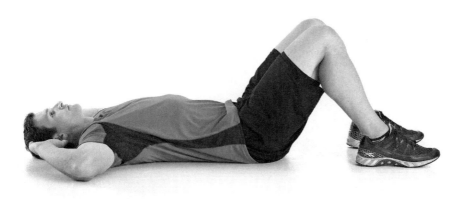

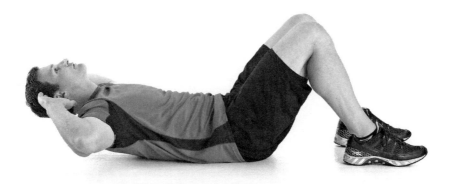

CRUNCH

Lie on your back with your knees bent and your hands behind your
ears. Slowly crunch up, bringing your shoulder blades off the ground.
Do as many crunches as you can.

DUMBBELL WORKOUT B

Dumbbell Thruster	8-12 reps
Walking Lunge	8-12 reps
Dumbbell Alternating Bench Press on Stability Ball	8-12 reps
Stability Ball Crunch	1 set to failure
Dumbbell Cross Punch	15-20 reps per arm
Corkscrew	1 set to failure

WORKOUT B

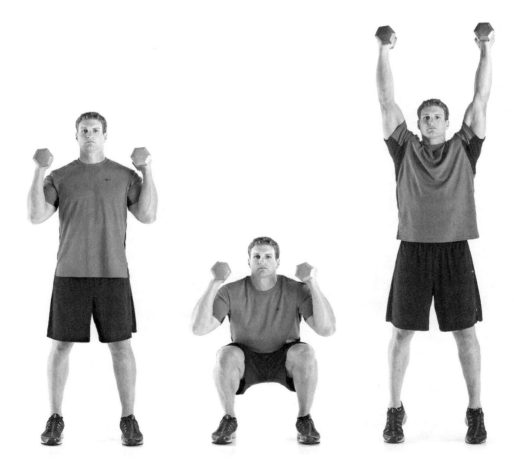

DUMBBELL THRUSTER

Grab a pair of dumbbells and hold them, arms bent, in front of your shoulders with palms facing each other. Position your feet shoulder-width apart, then quickly lower your hips until your thighs are parallel to the floor (or lower if you can). Explode back up and push the dumbbells above your head until your arms are straight. Pause, then lower the dumbbells as you squat back down and repeat.

WORKOUT **B**

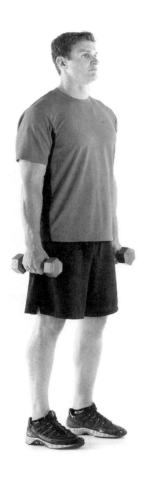

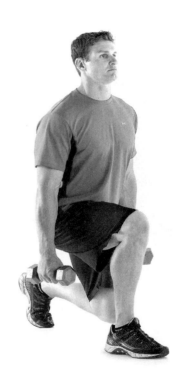

WALKING LUNGE

Grab a pair of dumbbells and hold them at your sides. Stand with your feet hip-width apart. Step forward with your right leg and slowly lower your body until your right knee is bent 90 degrees and your left knee nearly touches the floor. Your right lower leg should be perpendicular to the floor, and your torso should remain upright.

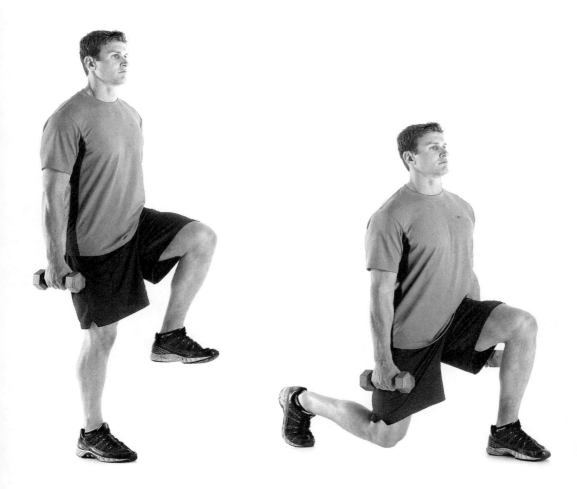

Pause momentarily, then push off your right leg and step forward
with your left leg so that your body is in the starting position again,
but a full lunge step ahead of where you began. (That's right, you'll
be walking forward with each lunge, so give yourself some room.)
Then repeat, lunging forward with your left leg. That's 1 repetition.
Do 8 to 12, alternating legs.

WORKOUT **B**

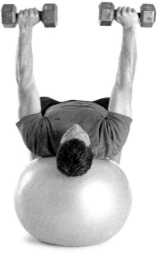

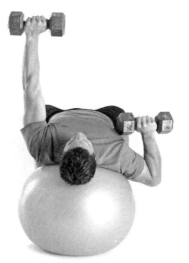

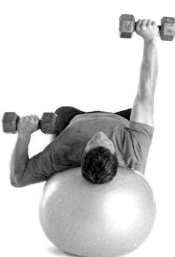

DUMBBELL ALTERNATING BENCH PRESS ON STABILITY BALL
As with a regular dumbbell bench press, get yourself into position
with your upper back, shoulders, and head supported by the ball and
your feet flat on the ground. Raise both dumbbells above you. Now,
lower one dumbbell to the bottom position and then drive it upward.
As you're driving the dumbbell up, simultaneously lower the other
dumbbell. Like two pistons in a car, your arms should be constantly
moving in an alternating fashion.

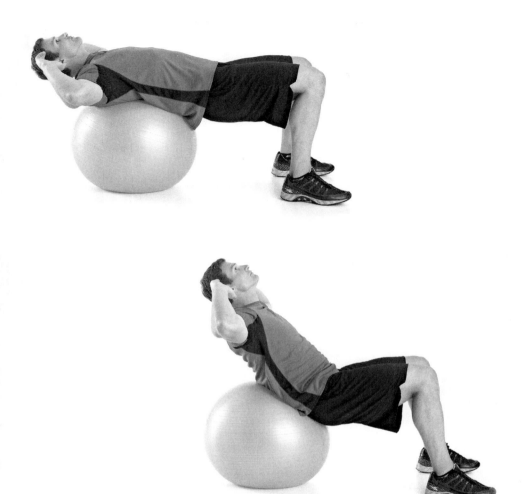

STABILITY BALL CRUNCH

Sit on a stability ball with your feet flat on the floor, shoulder width apart. Walk your feet forward as you lie back on the ball. Stop when the ball is under your hips, lower back, and middle back, knees bent 90 degrees. Your lower back should feel as if it is curved around the ball. Keep your head in line with your upper body. Place your hands behind your ears and draw in your abs. Raise your chest up and slightly forward in a crunching motion. Do not pull on your neck to initiate the crunch. You've reached the end of your range of motion when the middle of your back loses contact with the ball. Pause, slowly return to the starting position, then repeat. Do as many crunches as you can.

WORKOUT B

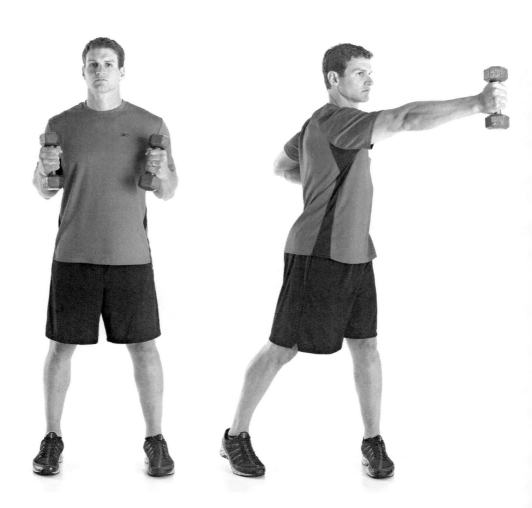

DUMBBELL CROSS PUNCH

Stand holding a pair of light dumbbells in front of you, palms facing in. Punch your right fist forward and to the left across your body, rotating your wrist as you go. Draw your arm back as you punch with your left fist. Perform 15 to 20 repetitions with each arm.

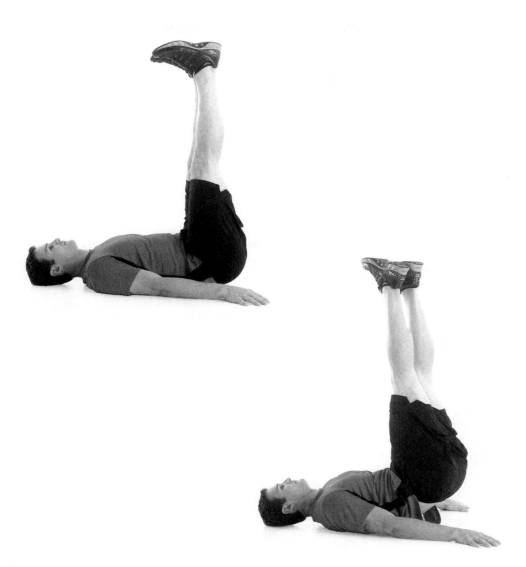

CORKSCREW

Lie on your back with your legs raised directly over your hips. Your knees should be slightly bent. Place your hands at your sides, palms down. Use your lower abs to raise your hips off the floor and toward your rib cage, elevating your feet straight up. Simultaneously twist your hips to the right. Hold for a second, and then return to the starting position. Repeat the exercise, this time twisting to the left.

POWER MOVES
16 Tricks to Get More from Your Workout

Over the years, we've collected some tweaks and tips from the best trainers and exercise physiologists in the nation. Here's a handful of our favorites for you to work into your workouts.

1. Smile when you stretch. It's hard to be tense when you are grinning. Try it. Letting all the tension out of your neck, shoulders, and arms will help you achieve a deeper, more effective stretch.

2. Try drop sets. Doing 5 reps or fewer per set with a weight that you can lift only five times trains your muscles to grow bigger and stronger, says Mark Peterson, an exercise and sport scientist at Arizona State University. Do 3 to 5 sets without rest, reducing the weight by 10 to 25 percent each set.

3. Never skip your crunches. After you bench-press, do 25 crunches on the bench. You'll be less likely to skip them than if you have to go find an exercise mat.

4. Change up your grip. It can help you do more repetitions. Try a set of barbell curls with a narrow grip. When you begin to fail, slide your hands out farther. You'll get more out of your biceps.

5. Use your legs for shoulder presses. Just a slight dip of the knees as you start each shoulder press will help you push more weight over your head. Your legs won't help you lower the load, so your shoulders reap the rewards.

6. Move the weight to the front during squats. It's easier to keep your back upright—and avoid injury—if you hold the weight across your chest, not behind your neck. This position also generates more power.

7. Use a mirror when lifting. It promotes better technique and helps prevent injury.

8. Add a shrug. Instead of lowering the weight at the top of a standing shoulder press, lock your elbows, pause, and shrug as if you were trying to touch your shoulders to your ears. Your trapezius and deltoids will benefit.

9. Never wait for a piece of exercise equipment. Your body is the best fitness tool you have. Next time a bench is bustling, add a set of pushups to your chest routine.

10. Stagger your squat stance every third workout. It will prevent your dominant leg from doing more than its share. Simply move one foot a few inches ahead of the other.

11. Take deeper, slower steps on the stairclimber. You'll burn more calories and work your leg muscles more fully than if you take short, choppy steps.

12. Go long. The longer your stride when running, the more effective your workout will be, according to University of Idaho researchers. They found that an extended stride length on cardio equipment can boost oxygen consumption by up to 12 percent and heart rate by 6 percent.

13. Flip your grip to become stronger instantly. At the National Strength and Conditioning Association's annual conference, scientists reported that men who performed the deadlift with an alternating grip—one hand grasping the bar overhand, the other underhand—could complete two more reps than when they used the traditional grip. As a result, the lifters hoisted an average of 713 more pounds each set.

14. If you suffer from sore shoulders, try this move from Tyler Wallace, CPT, of the National Academy of Sports Medicine, to strengthen your rotator cuffs: Attach a piece of resistance tubing to a sturdy support at waist level and stand with your left side toward the support. With your right hand, hold the tubing in front of your navel, with your elbow bent 90 degrees and your forearm parallel to the floor. Rotate your hand away from your body to a two-o'clock position, then return to the starting position. Do 2 or 3 sets of 12 to 15 with each arm.

15. Squeeze your knees. This move works your hamstrings and glutes, and will aid in preventing groin pulls, says Larry Brun, CSCS. Lie on your back with your knees bent 90 degrees and your feet flat on the floor. Place a stability ball between your knees. Lift your hips until only your heels, upper back, and head touch the floor. Pause, then lower your hips toward the floor without touching it, and repeat.

16. Finish your leg workout with walking lunges. Take large steps forward until the thigh of your front leg is parallel to the floor and the knee is over (not past) your toes.

REAL GUYS—REAL RESULTS

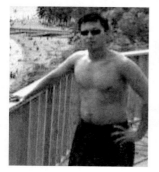

BEFORE:
208
POUNDS

AFTER:
165
POUNDS

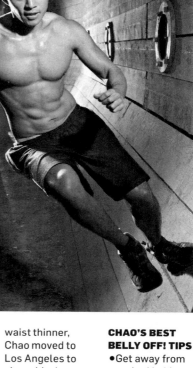

"Eating was a way for me to deal with stress."

VITALS: **Don Chao, 25, Los Angeles, CA**
OCCUPATION: **Actor/Wellness coach**
HEIGHT: **5'10"**
LESSON LEARNED: **Surround yourself with people who are as focused on fitness as you are.**

Chao sought refuge from the stress of college studies with a full-time party schedule. "I lifted weights three times a week," he says, "but I hit the keg and the junk food every night." His "earn your binges" attitude left him on the losing end of the transaction, with a layer of fat around his midsection.

THE TURNING POINT
After graduation, Chao spent a win-ter leading eco-tours in Brazil. He stopped snacking and eating carb-rich foods, switching to a diet of fish, chicken, and vegetables. He guided hikes along the Amazon, played soccer, did lots of pushups and pullups. In a few months, he uncovered his hidden lean physique.

LIFE IN THE FIT LANE
"When I came back from Brazil, I wanted to keep the weight off but gain muscle," he says. That meant loading up on protein—he takes in 150 grams of it a day in chicken, protein powder mixed with oatmeal, and meal replacement shakes. Now Chao visits the gym five times a week, working different muscle groups each day. On weekends, he runs mountain trails.

THE REWARD
With his head clear and his waist thinner, Chao moved to Los Angeles to chase his dream of being an actor. While his agent hunts for jobs, Chao works as a massage therapist and wellness coach, and spends a lot of time at the beach, where he noticed female heads turning his direction for a change. "I thought, 'so this is what it feels like to be checked out by a girl.'"

CHAO'S BEST BELLY OFF! TIPS
- Get away from your bad habits. Find your sanctuary for dodging temptation.
- Pay attention to your body after meals. Foods that make you feel bloated and tired will sap your energy during workouts.
- Make your mental fitness a priority. Visualizing your goal takes the same discipline as eating healthy.

BONUS SECTION: IGNITE YOUR FAT-BURNING FURNACE

Advanced Workouts for Faster Weight Loss

THE BODYWEIGHT AND DUMBBELL workouts in the earlier chapters of this book are ideal for the guy who's just starting out in a fitness routine or restarting one after a long layoff. By now you're past that point. You've built a solid base of fitness and are ready to take your fat-frying activity to the next level. And you may be ready to get back into the gym or start tossing around some substantial iron at home.

As you've already learned, muscle is the primary fat burner in your body. So the more of it you work, the faster you'll lose your gut. To engage the most muscle, spend time on exercises that hit your back, chest, gluteals, quadriceps, and hamstrings—the largest muscles you have. By training these major players, you'll also recruit the smaller muscles of your shoulders, arms, abs, and calves. The result: a total-body fat-burning workout.

SUPERSHOT
Double Your Gains

Adding a dumbbell row to a pushup will build your back as well as your chest, save time, and prevent muscle imbalances. Get into the classic pushup position but rest your hands on lightweight dumbbells. (Use hexagonal weights so they won't roll.) After doing a pushup, at the top position, pull one dumbbell off the floor, raising it to your chest until your elbow is above your back. Slowly return it to the floor and repeat with the other arm. Repeat the sequence.

In this chapter, we'll give you three advanced workouts that will test your mettle. The first workout is a classic power-lifting workout that utilizes just three exercises, and you can complete it in just 15 minutes. It's one of my all-time favorite workouts. When I played high school and college football, it was all that my lifting posse and I bothered with. It's efficient—perfect for those days when you want to push yourself hard but don't have an hour to spend in the gym. The second workout is a speedy circuit that splices aerobic exercise into resistance training moves. The third workout teams explosive moves with combination lifts to turbocharge your metabolism. Guys I see at the gym dig these routines because the versatility keeps workouts fresh and the specific moves within the routines bombard the muscles from many different angles. Try all of them during the next 6 to 8 weeks.

Finally, at the end of this chapter, you'll take the Belly Off! fitness test, a battery of five challenges that will measure your fitness level and provide you with instant feedback—motivation to keep pushing, keep burning fat, keep advancing toward your goal to get into the best shape of your life.

Are you ready? Let's go.

WORKOUT 1:
15-MINUTE POWER THREE

Research shows that lifting weights increases the rate at which your body burns fat for up to 48 hours after your workout. Not a bad payoff for a 15-minute commitment to hard, *really hard,* work.

This workout, a staple of power lifters, focuses on just three classic exercises—the barbell squat, the bench press, and the deadlift. These three moves work the major muscle groups for an incredibly efficient workout. But the key to getting the most from this trio is pushing yourself hard and using fairly heavy weight for the third set. You'll be huffing and puffing after each set—and the soreness in your muscles in the morning will remind you of how effective these moves are.

Warm up your muscles with the Belly Off! 2-Minute Drill, then jump right into the power three in this order: squats, bench press, and deadlift. Start with two light sets of 10 squat, resting for about 90 seconds in between. For the third set, load the barbell with a weight that you can lift only six times with your best effort. Perform a total of 5 reps using flawless form. Then rest for 2 minutes. Follow this same pattern—two light sets followed by a third heavy set—for the bench press and the deadlift. Ask someone to spot you, especially for the bench segment. Do this routine three times a week with a rest day in between—or as an emergency workout when you can't fit a longer one in at the gym.

EXERCISE	REPS
Barbell Squat	
Set 1	10 reps
REST	90 seconds
Set 2	10 reps
REST	90 seconds
Set 3	5 reps
REST	2 minutes
Bench Press	
Set 1	10 reps
REST	90 seconds
Set 2	10 reps
REST	90 seconds
Set 3	5 reps
REST	2 minutes
Deadlift	
Set 1	10 reps
REST	90 seconds
Set 2	10 reps
REST	90 seconds
Set 3	5 reps

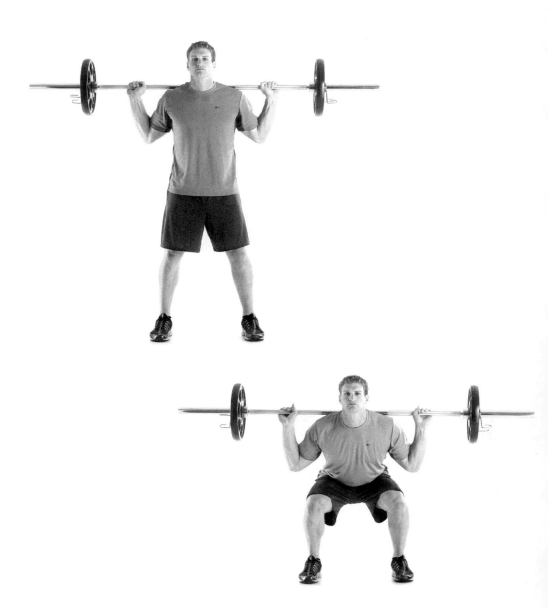

BARBELL SQUAT

Stand with your feet shoulder-width apart, and hold the barbell
across the back of your shoulders with an overhand grip. With your
back naturally arched, bend at the hips and knees until your thighs
are at least parallel to the floor. Then return to a standing position.

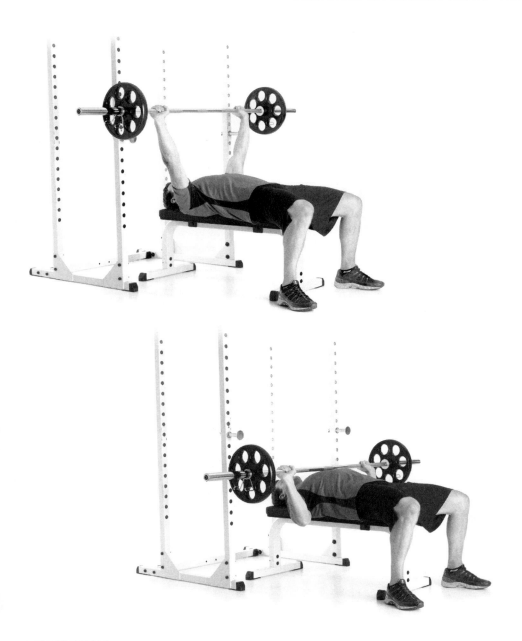

BENCH PRESS

Lie on a bench with your feet flat on the floor. Grab the bar with your hands more than shoulder-width apart, and hold it over your chest. Squeeze your shoulder blades down and together. As you lower the weight to your chest, pull your elbows toward your sides. Pause, then push the weight back up.

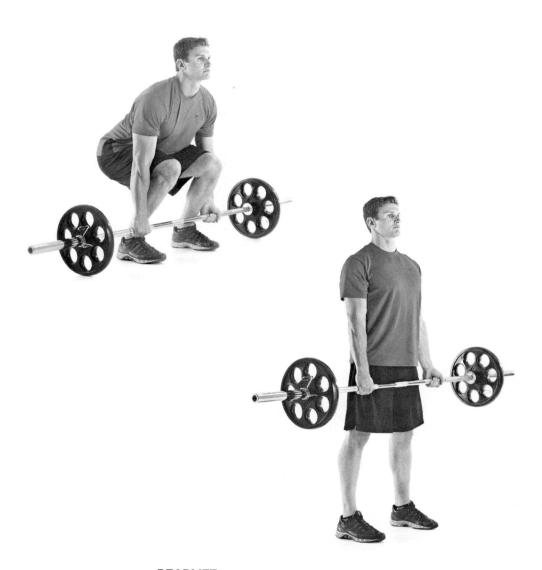

DEADLIFT

Stand with the bar on the floor in front of you so it just touches your shins. Push your hips back and grasp the bar with your hands just outside of your calves with an overhand grip. (I prefer an overhand grip for my right and an underhand grip for my left, as shown. It's a personal preference.) Keeping your back straight and chest up, drive your heels into the floor, and stand up. Then lower the bar back to the floor.

FAST AND FURIOUS CIRCUIT

Next time you are at the gym, observe your fellow sweat hogs—the men and the women. I've noticed that the women tend to be more efficient, moving methodically from exercise to exercise without, well, goofing off. I find that a lot of guys spend too much time sitting around between sets. They'll get a drink of water. Chat with their buds. Scribble into their workout charts. Check the newspaper. Watch CNN. Make time with the cutie at the juice bar. All that wastes minutes and leaves little time for cardiovascular exercise after the weight workout. So, this workout is designed to speed things up and eliminate that waste. Instead of rest periods after each set, you'll do short bursts of aerobic activity. You'll finish the workout faster and burn more calories as a result. Plus, doing exercises in a circuit this way—one after another without rest—adds an endurance component to strength training, which will improve your heart's ability to circulate oxygen to your muscles. This 4-week routine conditions all your major muscle groups with an emphasis on the lower body, which contains more than 50 percent of your body's muscle mass. Instead of resting between sets, do 30 to 45 seconds of cardio, such as jumping rope, jumping jacks, running on a treadmill, or riding a stationary bike.

Here's how to do it:

As always, begin by warming up with the Belly Off! 2-Minute Drill or about 5 minutes on the treadmill. Note: Unlike the classic trio workout, don't be concerned about the amount of weight you use in this one. Because you won't be resting, your muscles will fatigue faster than usual. So keep the weights fairly light. Start by doing this workout twice a week and gradually build up to three times a week, with rest days in between.

SUPERSHOT
Swim Out of Water

Lie chest down on a bench. Hold a $2\frac{1}{2}$-pound plate in each hand, arms straight in front of you. Keep one arm still and swing the other arm as if you were swimming freestyle. Alternate sets of 6 to 10 reps with each arm.

WEEK 1	WEEK 2	WEEK 3	WEEK 4
Choose one exercise from each of the four sections below (A, B, C, and D).	**Do** the four moves you didn't do last week.	**Do** both moves in sections A, B, C, and D.	**Do** both moves in sections A, B, C, and D.
Do 3 sets of each exercise, 10 to 12 reps each.	**Do** 3 sets of each exercise, 12 to 15 reps each.	**Do** 2 sets of each exercise for a total of 16 sets.	**Do** 2 sets of each exercise for a total of 16 sets.
Don't rest between sets. Your workout will total 12 sets.	**Don't** rest between sets. Your workout will total 12 sets.	**Do** 12 to 15 repetitions per set.	**Do** 15 to 20 repetitions per set.
		Don't rest between sets. Do this workout two or three times a week.	**Don't** rest between sets. Do this workout two or three times a week.

SECTION A	SECTION B	SECTION C	SECTION D
Deadlift	Ranging-Stance Squat	Clean and Press	Varied-Level Bench Press
Single-Leg Bent-Over Row	Ratchet Leg Press	Push Press	Single-Arm Rotational Chest Press

SECTION A

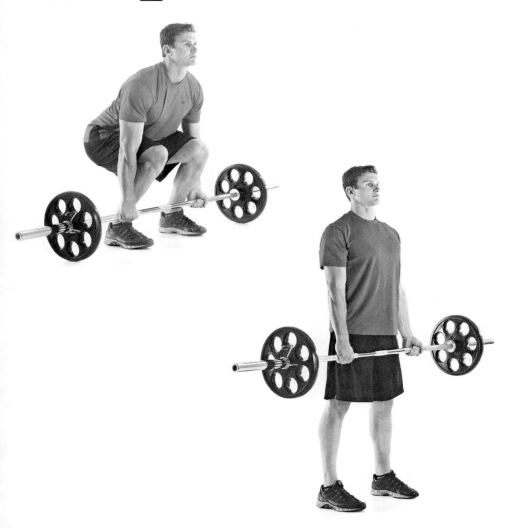

DEADLIFT

Stand with a barbell on the floor in front of you, with the bar over your toes. Bend your knees and grasp the bar with an overhand grip, your hands just outside your knees. Keeping your head and back straight, slowly stand up, keeping the bar close to your body as you lift, until your legs are straight. Pause, then slowly lower the bar to the floor.

Tip: Avoid rounding your lower back, which increases your risk of a herniated disk.

SECTION **A**

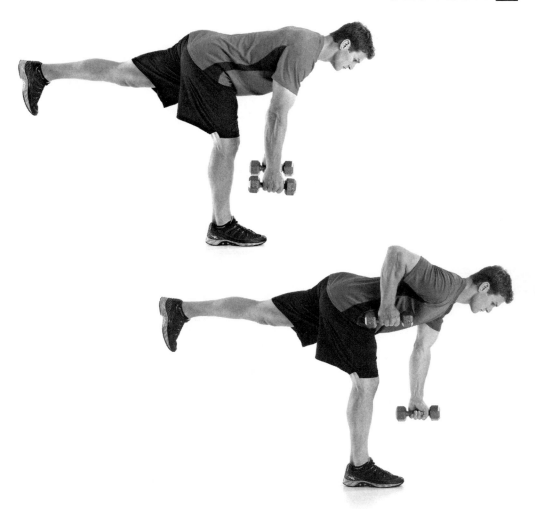

SINGLE-LEG BENT-OVER ROW

Stand on one foot holding a pair of dumbbells with your arms hanging in front of you. Bend forward at the waist until your back is almost parallel to the floor and raise your other leg behind you. Now pull the weight in your right hand to the right side of your chest. As you lower it, bring the weight in your left hand to the left side of your chest. That's 1 rep. Continue alternating arms for 5–6 reps, then switch legs and repeat.

Tip: If you can't maintain balance, try raising and lowering both weights together.

SECTION B

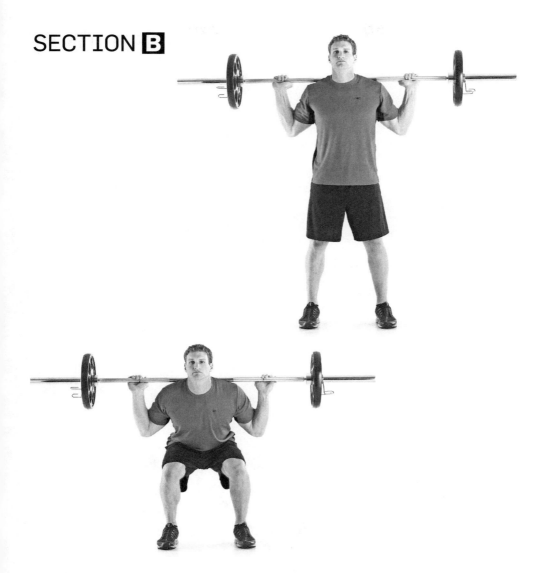

RANGING-STANCE SQUAT

Place a barbell across the back of your shoulders and stand with your feet shoulder-width apart. Keeping your back straight, lower your body until your thighs are at least parallel to the floor. Pause, then push yourself back up and repeat until you've completed 1 set. Do the second set with your feet spaced 2 inches wider than shoulder-width apart. Place them another 2 inches apart for the third set.

Tip: If spreading your feet wide feels awkward, try turning your toes slightly outward before you start your set.

SECTION B

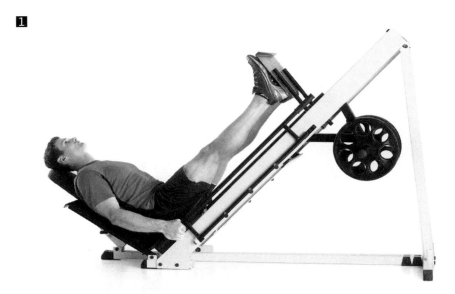

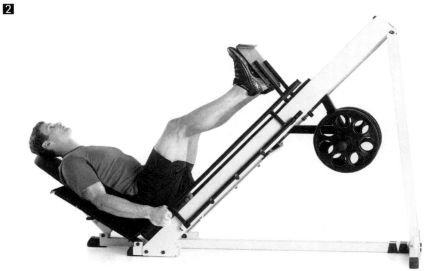

RATCHET LEG PRESS

(1) Sit in a leg-press machine with your back against the pad and your feet hip-width apart on the platform. Press the weight up until your legs are straight, knees unlocked. (2) Slowly lower the weight a few inches, pause for a second, (3) then lower it another few inches

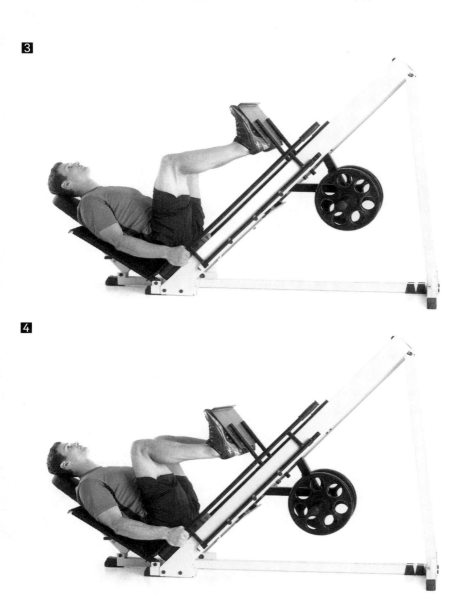

and (4) pause again. Continue this stop-and-start technique until your legs are bent 90 degrees, then push the weight back up until your legs are straight. That's 1 repetition.

Tip: Perform the move slowly for a better lift.

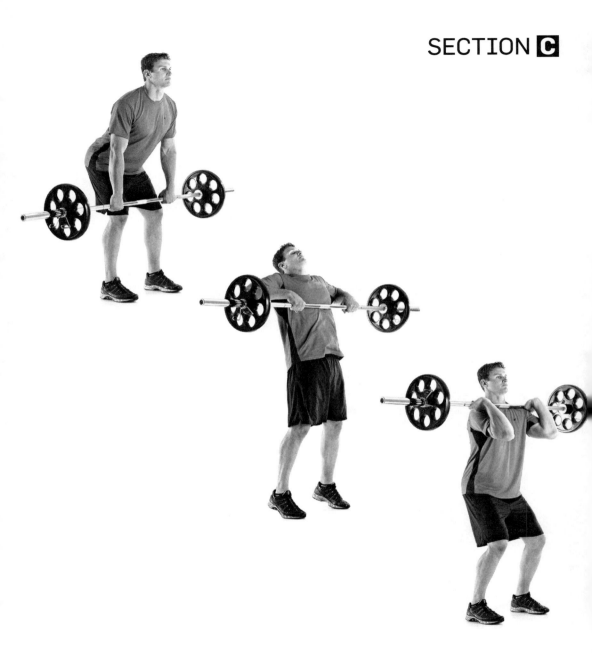

CLEAN AND PRESS

Stand holding a barbell in front of you, hands and feet shoulder-width apart. Bend your knees slightly and lean forward so the bar hangs at your knees. Now quickly explode up as if you were jumping and trying to throw the bar overhead. As you rise on the balls of your feet, shrug your shoulders, pull the bar up to shoulder level, and dip down with

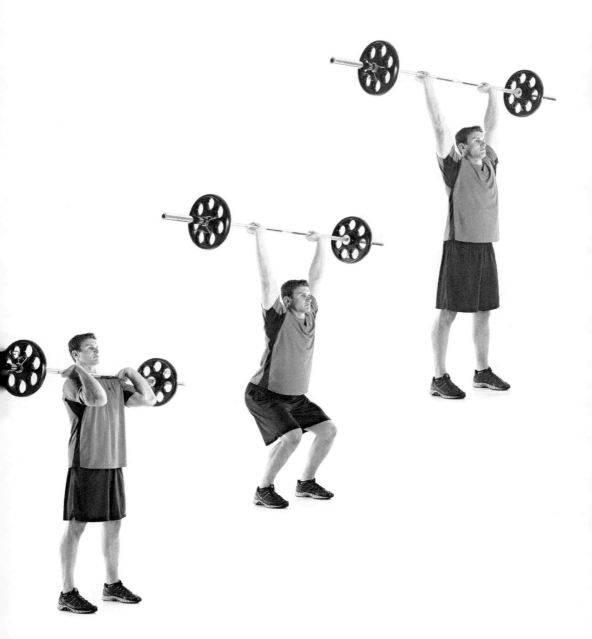

your knees to "catch" the bar on your shoulders. Straighten your legs. Press the weight overhead while bending your knees. Stand straight up with the bar overhead, then return to the starting position.

Tip: Don't stop and start between parts of the exercise.

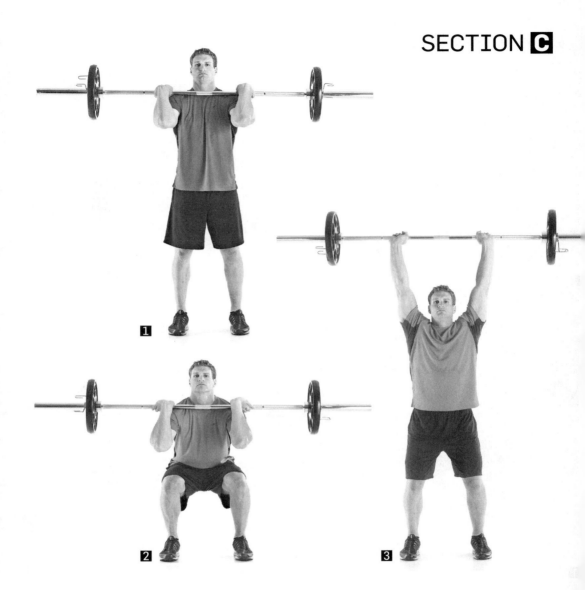

PUSH PRESS

(1) Stand with a barbell across the front of your shoulders, hands slightly wider than shoulder-width apart, elbows pointing forward. (You can load the barbell with more weight than you normally would for a shoulder press.) (2) Bend your knees and lower your body a few inches, (3) then quickly push back up as you thrust the weight overhead. Lower the weight to the front of your shoulders.

Tip: Use your legs. The momentum you'll create by squatting should allow you to use heavier weights for bigger results.

SECTION **D**

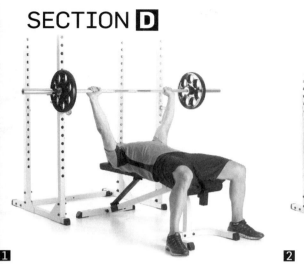
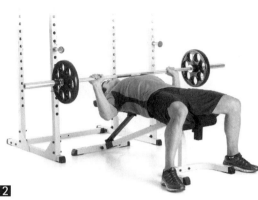

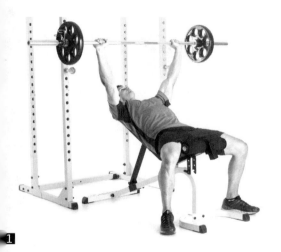
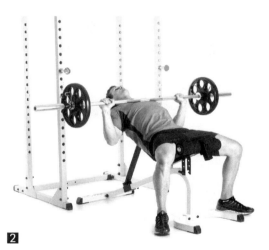

VARIED-LEVEL BENCH PRESS

Lie on an adjustable weight bench and grab the bar with your hands shoulder-width apart and your feet flat on the floor. (1) Lift the bar off the supports and hold it above your chest. Slowly lower the bar to your chest (2), then press it up and slightly back. For each additional set, raise the bench one notch (or about a 10- to 15-degree incline).

Tip: Lower the bar to a point on your chest that's just above your nipples. If it strays below that spot, it can put too much strain on your rotator-cuff muscles.

SECTION D

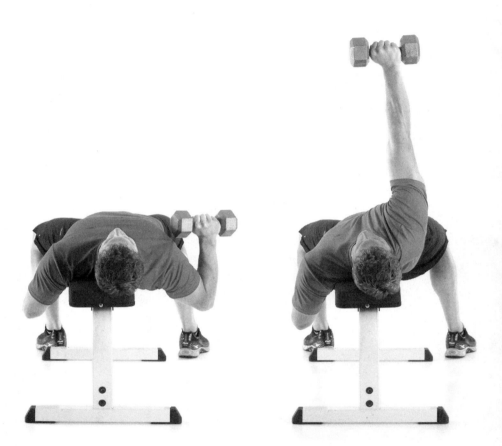

SINGLE-ARM ROTATIONAL CHEST PRESS

Lie on a bench holding a dumbbell in your right hand, next to your chest. Slide your body to the right so your right side hangs off the bench. (Grab the left side of the bench with your left hand for balance.) Press the weight up and lift your right shoulder as high as you can, then lower the weight. Switch positions and use your other hand for the next set.

Tip: Your shoulder blade can rise off the bench at the top of the move, but keep your head flat against the bench.

EXPLOSIVE COMBOS

Like the last circuit, the fast pace of this routine melts fat and boosts endurance. This will help you eventually go harder and longer—to get leaner faster. What's unique about this workout routine is that it is designed to engage more muscles than typical body-building routines do. And that means you'll burn more calories than ever before. Take, for example, the traveling deadlift (page 162) and the extremely challenging Turkish getup (page 158)—both require balance and stamina. Plus, this workout incorporates power exercises, such as the hang clean and the jump squat, which target your fast-twitch muscle fibers. These fibers have the greatest potential for size and strength gains, which translates to greater fat burn.

A recent study from the University of Southern Maine found that an intense weight-training session burns as many as 71 percent more calories than previously thought—putting it on par with aerobic exercise. Explosive moves, also known as plyometrics, are terrific training for all sorts of competitive sports, such as basketball, football, soccer, and tennis.

The following workout plan creates an enormous metabolic demand on your body by blending explosive exercises and combination lifts in a fast-paced circuit. Alternate between Workout A and Workout B, performing three workouts a week and resting a day between sessions. During the first 2 weeks, do 3 sets of each exercise, resting 60 seconds between sets. During Weeks 3 and 4, perform each routine as a circuit. That is, do 1 set of each exercise without resting between moves, then rest 90 seconds between circuits. Complete a total of three circuits.

WORKOUT A

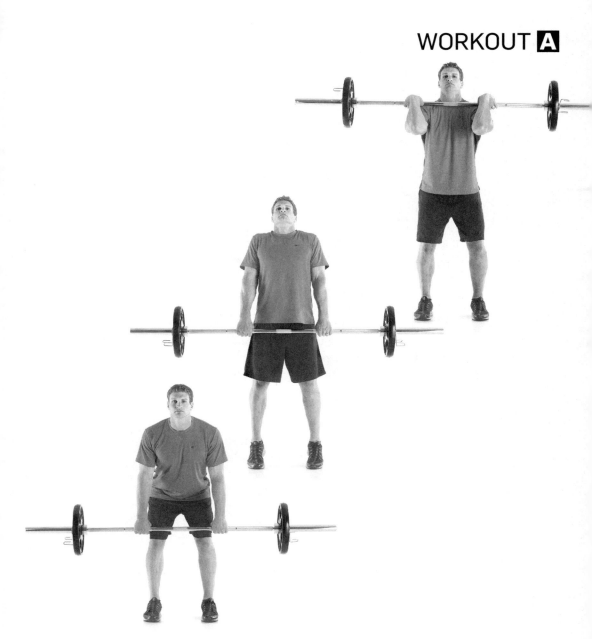

HANG CLEAN TO FRONT SQUAT TO PUSH PRESS

Grab a barbell with a shoulder-width grip and dip your knees, as if
you were about to jump. Quickly reverse the motion and shrug your
shoulders as you pull the bar straight up and rise onto your toes. As
the bar approaches chest height, bend your knees and swing your
elbows forward to "catch" the bar in the crooks of your fingers.

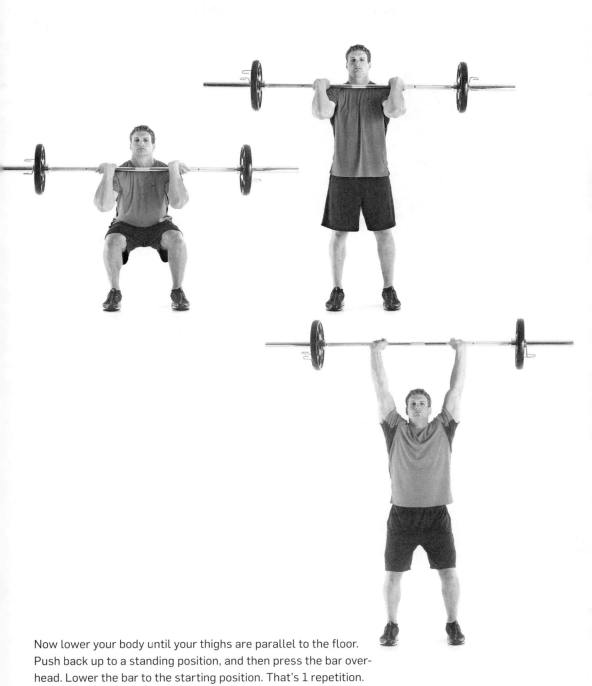

Now lower your body until your thighs are parallel to the floor. Push back up to a standing position, and then press the bar overhead. Lower the bar to the starting position. That's 1 repetition.

Do 6 repetitions with a weight you would typically use to push press six times.

WORKOUT A

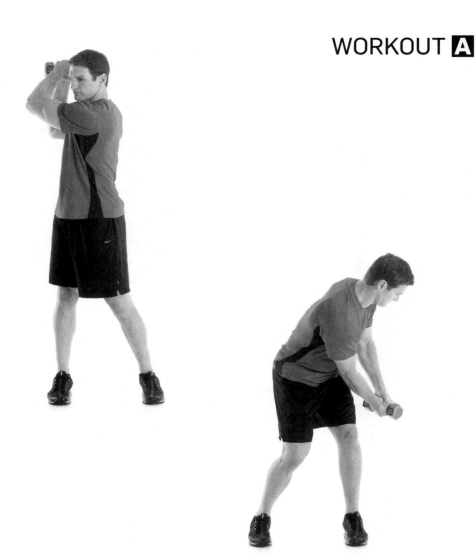

DUMBBELL DOUBLE WOOD CHOP

Hold a light dumbbell with two hands, your arms extended above your right shoulder. Keeping your arms straight but not locked, bend at the knees and forcefully rotate your torso to the left as you draw your arms down and across your body. When your hands reach the outside of your left knee, pause, then quickly reverse the movement with the same intensity, pausing at the top. That's 1 repetition. Do 8 reps, then hold the weight over your left shoulder and repeat the move, this time chopping to your right. Complete 8 repetitions on each side.

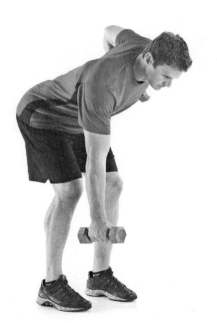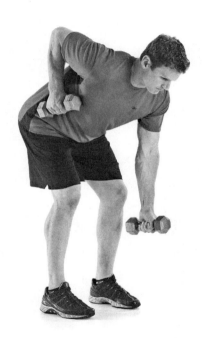

PISTON BENT-OVER ROW

Holding dumbbells, stand with your feet shoulder-width apart. Bend forward until your torso is almost parallel to the floor and your arms hang straight down, palms facing each other. Pull the weights to the sides of your chest. This is the starting position. Keeping your left arm as still as possible, lower the weight in your right hand until your arm is straight. Lift the dumbbell back up to the side of your chest, while simultaneously lowering your left hand. Continue alternating. Complete 8 repetitions with each arm.

WORKOUT **A**

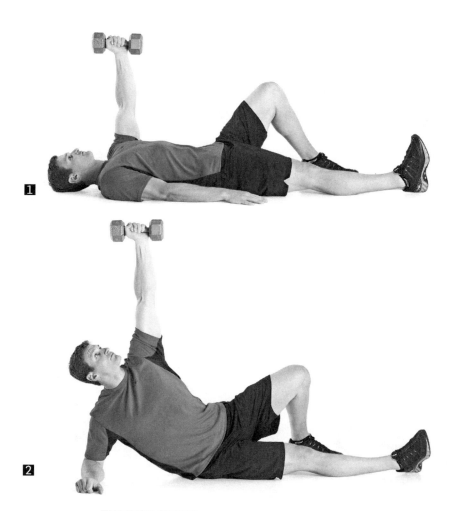

1

2

TURKISH GETUP

(1) Lie on your back with your right leg straight and your left leg bent. Hold a light dumbbell in your left hand with your arm straight above you. Keeping your elbow locked and the weight above you at all times, move your legs and right arm underneath you to push yourself up to a standing position (2–5). Still keeping your left arm straight and the weight above you, reverse the motion to return to the starting position. Do 8 repetitions on each side.

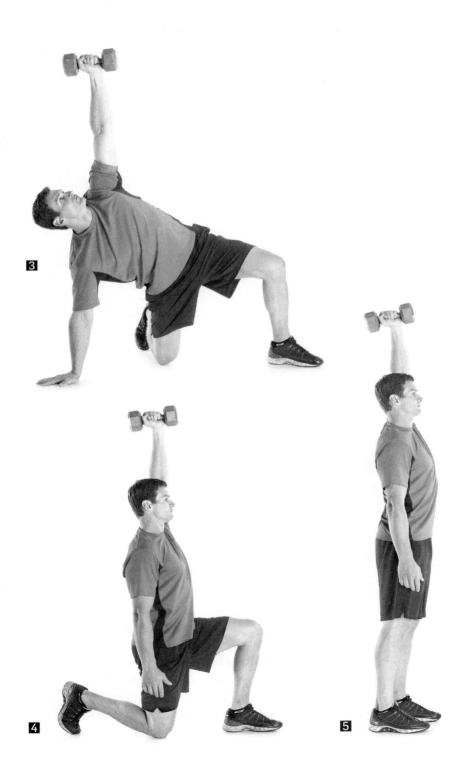

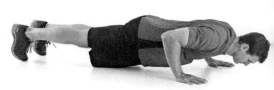

WORKOUT B

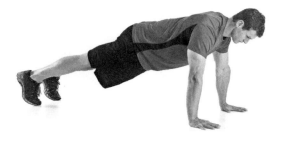

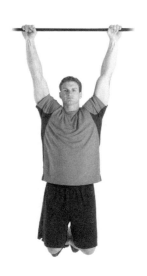

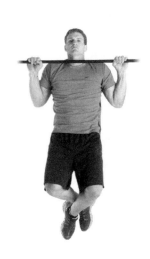

PUSHUP/PULLUP LADDER

Stand next to a pullup bar and get into pushup position. Do 2 pushups, then stand up and grasp the bar with your hands slightly more than shoulder-width apart. Pull yourself up until the bar is at shoulder height, then lower yourself. Add 2 pushups and 1 pullup each time you repeat the pair. So you'll start by doing 2 pushups and 1 pullup. Next, you'll do 4 and 2, then 6 and 3, and so on until you can do 10 pushups and 5 pullups or until you can't do any more with proper form. Perform 3 ladders in Weeks 1 and 2; do the ladder as part of a circuit in Weeks 3 and 4.

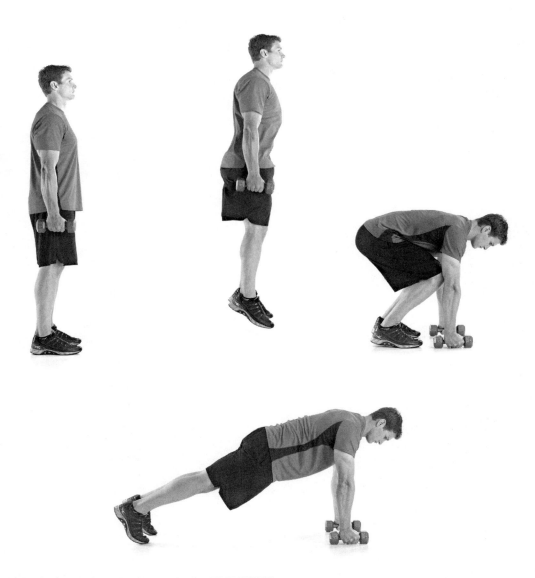

DUMBBELL JUMP SQUAT TO SQUAT THRUST

Stand with your feet shoulder-width apart and hold a pair of dumbbells at your sides. Lower your body about 6 inches, then jump as
high as you can. Land softly on the balls of your feet and immediately sink into a squat, lowering your body until you touch the
dumbbells to the floor. Kick your legs out behind you so you're in a
pushup position, with your hands on top of the dumbbells. Reverse
the motion, bringing your legs forward so your feet are under your
shoulders, then pushing back up to a standing position. That's 1
repetition. Do 8 repetitions.

WORKOUT B

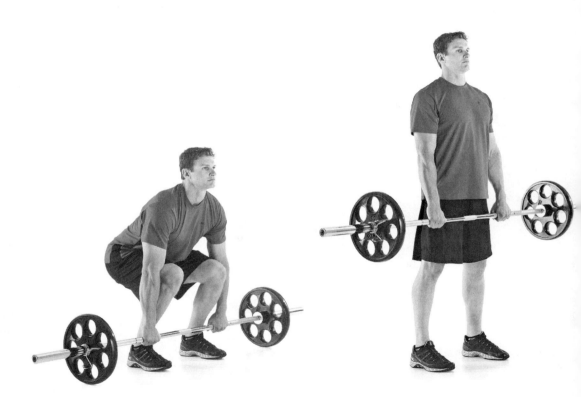

TRAVELING DEADLIFT

Stand with a light barbell on the floor in front of you, your feet shoulder-width apart and the bar directly over your toes. Bend your knees and grasp the bar with an overhand grip with your hands just outside of your knees. Keeping your head and back straight and the

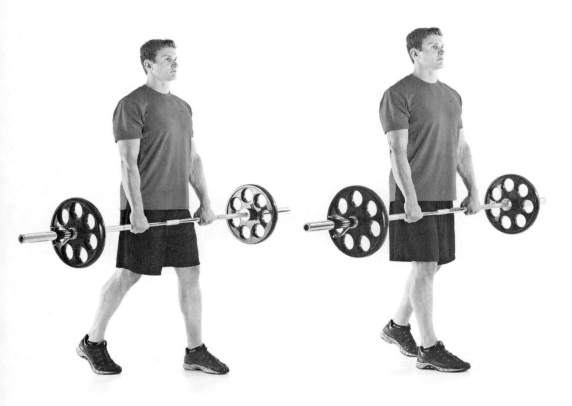

bar close to your body, stand up. Next, step forward with your left
foot and then with your right so your feet come together. Lower the
bar to the floor and repeat the move, this time stepping forward with
your right foot. Do 8 to 10 repetitions.

WORKOUT B

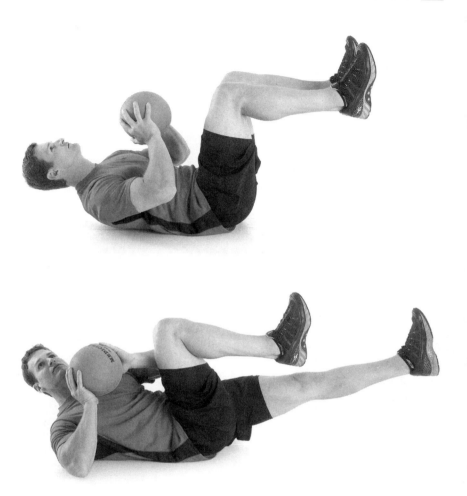

MEDICINE-BALL BICYCLES

Lie on your back holding a medicine ball in front of your chest,
elbows flared out to the sides. Bend your knees 90 degrees and
raise your legs so your thighs are perpendicular to the floor. Next,
curl your torso up so your shoulders are off the floor. This is the
starting position. Bring your right knee toward your chest as you
straighten your left leg, and simultaneously twist your upper body
to the right until your left elbow meets your right knee. Reverse the
move, drawing your left knee to your right elbow. Do 10 repetitions
on each side.

SPINNING INTERVAL

You can do this interval workout on a stationary bicycle or spinning cycle at home or at the gym. It'll take you about 30 minutes. Keep a water bottle handy. You're going to need it.

Clip in, start pedaling, and follow this sequence:

Warmup: 1 minute of easy pedaling
1 minute: climb, increase resistance but stay in the saddle
1 minute: climb, stand up out of the saddle
1 minute: recovery, reduce resistance, sit down and pedal easily
2 minutes: climb, in the saddle, increase resistance to simulate a hill
2 minutes: climb, out of the saddle, increase resistance and pedal while standing
2 minutes: recovery, reduce resistance, seated
3 minutes: climb, in the saddle, increase resistance
3 minutes: climb, out of the saddle, increase resistance
2 minutes: recovery, reduce resistance, seated
15 seconds: fast pedaling, seated, more resistance
15 seconds: recovery, reduce resistance, seated
15 seconds: fast pedaling, seated
15 seconds: recovery, slower pedaling, seated
15 seconds: fast pedaling, seated
15 seconds: recovery, slower pedaling, seated
15 seconds: fast pedaling, seated
15 seconds: recovery, slower pedaling, seated
30 seconds: fast pedaling, seated
30 seconds: recovery, slower pedaling, seated
30 seconds: fast pedaling, seated
30 seconds: recovery, slower pedaling, seated
1 minute: fast pedaling, seated
1 minute: recovery, slower pedaling, seated
32 counts: fast pedaling out of the saddle
32 counts: fast pedaling in the saddle
16 counts: fast pedaling out of the saddle
16 counts: fast pedaling in the saddle
8 counts: fast pedaling out of the saddle
8 counts: fast pedaling in the saddle
Cooldown: 1 minute of easy pedaling

HOW FIT ARE YOU?
Take This 5-Exercise Test to Find Out

If you are like most men I know, you're pretty competitive. You like to know how you measure up against other guys and how you're doing this week versus last week. The following fitness test is a great way to gauge the progress you've made on the Belly Off! Diet. It'll motivate you to keep going and try to better your score the next time. I recommend you do this five-point challenge after the first 4 weeks of the program and once a month thereafter, keeping track of your scores. The test gauges your ability in five performance standards. See how you measure up, then improve with our advanced Belly Off! Club training programs at www.menshealth.com/bellyoff.

THE VERTICAL JUMP TEST
Demonstrates your explosive power and overall athletic ability

HOW TO DO IT: Stand facing a wall, extend one arm up, and mark your reach with chalk. Then jump as high as you can with the chalk in your hand and make another mark at the highest point. The space between marks is your vertical jump.

RATINGS:
Out of shape: < 16 inches
Average: 16–18 inches
Fit: 19–24 inches
Belly Off! fit: > 24 inches

THE 1-MILE CHALLENGE
A measuring stick of stamina and determination since grade school. A 6-minute mile remains the mark of a fit man.

HOW TO DO IT: Go to a high school track. Set your stopwatch and go.

RATINGS:
Out of shape: 10 minutes or more
Average: 8–9 minutes
Fit: 7 minutes
Belly Off! fit: 6 minutes or less

THE CHINUP CHALLENGE
Measures the strength and endurance of one of your largest muscle groups—your back.

HOW TO DO IT: Start from a full hang, hands shoulder-width apart, palms toward you. Pull your chin over the bar, and then lower your body back down.

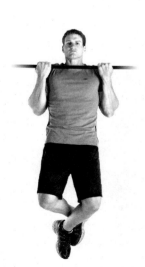

RATINGS:
Out of shape: 0 reps
Average: 1–4 reps
Fit: 5–8 reps
Belly Off! fit: 9 reps or more

THE SINGLE-LEG SQUAT TEST

Not only does it test leg strength, but this exercise requires tremendous core control.

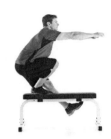

HOW TO DO IT: Stand on a bench. Hold your arms in front of you and flex your left ankle so your toes point up. Keeping your torso as upright as possible, bend your right knee and slowly lower your body until your left heel touches the floor. Pause 1 second, then push yourself up. That's 1 repetition.

RATINGS:
Out of shape: 0 reps
Average: 1 rep
Fit: 2–4 reps
Belly Off! fit: 5 reps or more

THE PUSHUP TEST

Gauges the amount of force you're able to generate with your chest, triceps, and shoulders while staying strong throughout your body's core.

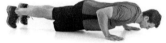

HOW TO DO IT: Assume the classic pushup position: legs straight, hands beneath your shoulders. Brace your abs.
Keeping your body rigid, lower yourself until your chest touches the floor. Then push back up until your arms are extended.

RATINGS:
Out of shape: < 20 reps
Average: 20–34 reps
Fit: 35–49 reps
Belly Off! fit: > 49 reps

PART III

The Belly Off! Diet
Real Meal Plan

7

EAT WELL WHILE FIGHTING FLAB

Easy Recipes, Simple Shopping Lists, Guy Foods That Taste Great

EATING IS ONE OF LIFE'S supreme joys. I know I'm not going to get any argument here. But think about how delightful it is to tuck into a slab of baby back ribs slathered in barbecue sauce or a masterfully grilled tuna steak. To crunch into a crisp garden salad drizzled with extra-virgin olive oil and balsamic vinegar. Or cut into the perfect veal chop.

Life should be about eating that way. Eating well. And savoring every bite. You don't want to deny yourself the pleasure of eating good food. Yet most diets ask you to do just that. Many are about sacrificing what you love to eat. And that has a lot to do with why those diets are destined for failure. Diets that force you to deny yourself your favorite foods are virtually impossible to follow for any length of time. Having willpower is, well, empowering, but sacrificing can be extreme and ultimately too difficult for most.

The *Men's Health* philosophy is this: We strongly believe that if you make smart choices from a variety of food groups, exercise practical portion control, and break a sweat most days of the week, you can generally eat whatever you wish. We understand that we're human. We're men. We get hungry. Flavor and satisfaction are important to us. And when we've done a good job at whatever it is that we do, we deserve a good meal. Unless your doctor demands it, there's really no reason that you should have to stop eating steak or Chinese food, or go cold turkey on pizza. They aren't the dietary devils they've been made out to be. It's how we eat them and how much of them we eat that can cause us trouble. It's those bad choices we're making—heavy on the processed foods and sugary and calorie-laden snacks—that put on the pounds.

On the following pages, you'll find recipes for the Belly Off! Diet Real Meals. These are traditional guy-food favorites for breakfast, lunch, and dinner. We didn't select them because they're ultra low in fat or carbohydrates or calories. If we did, you wouldn't eat them—because they'd taste like kitty litter. We did, however, take a *reasonable* approach to calories, carbohydrates, fat, and protein, and we kept a keen eye on portion size. (You've got to help us here.) Whenever possible, we suggest recipes that prepare one serving to help you avoid overeating. In some cases—like casseroles, stews, soups, salads, and steak dinners—it's not practical (or economical) to make just one serving. Use these meals to share with family or a friend. Or wrap up the leftovers for another meal at home or to take to work for lunch.

All these meals taste good. I've tried them. And they're easy to prepare, too. That's important. Recipes with too many steps or too many ingredients and pots and pans turn me off. And I'm guessing that you appreciate simpler-is-better, too. I'm a fairly decent cook now—thanks to my wife's tutoring. When I was single, however, my dinners were

IT WORKS FOR ME

"When I go out at night with friends or my rugby team, I make sure to eat some protein, like slices of turkey wrapped around a piece of cheese— before leaving home. That fills me up so I'm not tempted by high-calorie snacks."

—Ben Lewis, Chicago, who lost 11 pounds in his first 2 weeks on the Belly Off! Diet

no-brainer meals: fried hamburgers, instant white rice with a can of red beets dumped over it, boxed mac 'n' cheese—you know, with that orange, powdered, cheesy substance you mix with milk and margarine.

I can't believe I cooked that way, but I did. No wonder I ate out a lot. I was living in Dallas, so that meant Tex-Mex or barbecue four or five nights a week. At least once a week for lunch, we'd head over to Sonny Bryan's Smokehouse at the corner of Inwood and Harry Hines, order pulled pork or sliced beef sandwiches with extra sauce, Texas onion rings, and Dr. Peppers, and eat on the hood of the car. On the weekends, at a football game or rodeo, it wasn't unusual to grab a Frito pie for a snack. For you Yankees, that's an open bag of Fritos corn chips into which you dump chopped onions, grated Cheddar cheese, and a ladle of chili (without beans).

Even when my friends and I got together to grill healthy fajitas and eat them with red beans and rice, we'd overdo it on the tortilla chips *con queso* and *cerveza*. A couple of years of eating that way added girth to my gut and sent my cholesterol soaring over the 250 mark. Then, one day while picking up my canned beets at the Tom Thumb grocery store on Belt Line Road in Irving, Texas, I spotted a new magazine I had never seen before. It was called *Men's Health*; and in it I found an article on natural ways to lower cholesterol, plus a low-fat turkey and bean chili recipe that was easy enough for a klutz like me to make. I bought the magazine and the chili ingredients and went back to my apartment to make the meal. I was hooked on both the recipe and the magazine. In fact, after I finished reading, I immediately sent my resume to the editor. A couple of months later, I made my way north to Pennsylvania to work at *Men's Health* as a senior editor writing about fitness and weight loss. That was in 1992. And I'm still using that same turkey chili recipe today.

Here it is. Enjoy. And don't forget the Tabasco.

SUPERSHOT
Add Flavor,
Cut Calories

Instead of slathering butter on your corn on the cob, squeeze some lemon juice over the corn and sprinkle on garlic powder or Old Bay Seasoning. You'll save about 100 calories.

Men's Health One-Pot Turkey Chili

1	large onion, chopped
1	large orange, red, or yellow bell pepper, chopped
1	clove garlic, minced
1½	pounds lean ground turkey breast
1	can (28-ounces) diced tomatoes
1	can (15 ounces) no-salt-added tomato sauce
1	can (15 ounces) red kidney beans, rinsed and drained
1	can (15 ounces) pinto beans, rinsed and drained
1–2	tablespoons chili powder to taste
1	teaspoon ground cumin
¼	teaspoon red pepper flakes
½	cup reduced-fat sour cream
½	cup shredded reduced-fat Cheddar cheese

1. Add olive oil to a large pot or Dutch oven, and sauté onions, bell pepper, and garlic over medium-high heat. Dump in the turkey and break up with a wooden spoon while cooking for 5 minutes, or until all the turkey turns white (no longer pink). Stir in the tomatoes with their juice, tomato sauce, kidney beans, pinto beans, chili powder, cumin, and red pepper flakes. Bring to a boil on medium-high heat.

2. Cover, turn down the heat to medium-low, and cook on medium for 1 to 1½ hours.

3. Ladle into bowls, topping each serving with 1 tablespoon of sour cream and 1 tablespoon of the shredded cheese. Add a couple of dashes of Tabasco sauce. And maybe a few pickled jalapeno slices.

MAKES 6 TO 8 SERVINGS.

Per serving (based on 6 servings): 299 calories, 30 g protein, 31 g carbohydrates, 6 g fat (2.7 g saturated), 8 g fiber

Chapter 4 gave you a very detailed and prescriptive meal plan for every day. The purpose was to make you familiar with the meals, offer a variety of tastes, and get you into the habit of eating more frequently. You get the picture now. And you don't need me telling you to eat chicken tonight when you feel like eating beef. Still, you might appreciate some suggestions for meal planning. So, here you get just that—a selection of five meals for breakfasts, lunches, and dinners for each of the next 3 weeks. You can mix them up as you like, and what you eat on the other 2 days of the week is entirely up to you as long as it follows the Belly Off! Diet principles. The idea is to give you a basic plan to build upon. And a shopping list for the planned meals each week to make your life easier.

WEEK 2 SUGGESTED MEALS

BREAKFASTS	LUNCHES	DINNERS
American-English Egg Sandwich (page 178)	Mediterranean Wrap (page 184)	One-Pot Chicken Pasta with a Kick (page 191)
Quick Thick Yogurt with Extras (page 179)	Leftover chicken pasta (page 191)	Blue-Plate Special Meatloaf (page 193) with Better-for-You Fries (page 196)
Huevos Rancheros Wrap with Canadian bacon (page 179)	Turkey-Avocado Cobb Salad (page 185)	Mediterranean-Style Cod (page 210)
Kashi Honey Sunshine whole-grain cereal	Belly Off! Pizza with The Works (page 187)	BBQ Beer Ribs (page 196)
Chocolate Power Oatmeal (page 183)	Peanut butter and preserves sandwich	Cedar-Plank Salmon (page 213)

WEEK 2 SHOPPING LIST

DAIRY			
blue cheese	low-fat American cheese	Parmesan cheese	reduced-fat Mexican
eggs	low-fat blueberry yogurt	1% or fat-free milk	blend cheese
fat-free egg substitute	mozzarella cheese		

FRUITS AND VEGETABLES			
alfalfa sprouts	basil leaves	fennel	plum tomatoes
apples	broccoli	fresh or frozen blueberries	red onion
asparagus	button mushrooms	mint leaves	scallions
avocado	celery	onions	zucchini
baby spinach	cherry tomatoes	oranges	
baking potatoes	cilantro	orange, red, yellow, and	
bananas	English cucumber	green bell peppers	

BREADS, CEREALS, AND PASTAS			
Barilla Plus multigrain penne pasta	brown rice	oat bran	whole-wheat English muffins
Boboli 100% Whole Wheat pizza crust	Kashi Honey Sunshine whole-grain cereal	rolled oats	whole-wheat tortillas
	low-fat granola	whole-wheat bread	

MEATS AND FISH			
8 boneless country-style pork ribs	Canadian bacon	ground turkey breast	turkey bacon
boneless, skinless chicken breast	2 cod fillets	salmon fillets	turkey breast cutlets
	extra-lean ground beef		

OTHER			
chili sauce	extra-virgin olive oil	minced ginger	slivered almonds
chocolate whey protein powder	flaxseeds	onion flakes	spicy tomato juice cocktail
cider vinegar	garlic	prepared olive tapanade	sun-dried tomatoes
Dijon mustard	Heinz One-Carb ketchup	rosemary	sun-dried tomato pesto
dried mustard	honey barbecue sauce	salsa	thyme
	hummus	sesame seeds	tomato paste

WEEK 3 SUGGESTED MEALS

BREAKFASTS	LUNCHES	DINNERS
Quick and Healthy Oatmeal (page 183)	Cold Hot Tuna Sandwich (page 188)	Grilled Spicy Fish Tacos (page 212)
Easy, Cheesy Breakfast Burrito (page 181)	Chipotle Turkey Burger (page 206)	Frank's Flank Steak (page 198)
Kashi Honey Sunshine cereal	Eat-It-Cold Shrimp and Pasta Salad (page 186)	Shrimp Fra Diavolo (page 205)
Protein Oatmeal Powerboost (page 180)	Leftover flank steak (page 198)	Blackened Snapper with Mango Salsa (page 204)
Hill Country Omelet (page 182)	Cheese 'n' Chili Chicken (page 202)	Maple Mustard Pork Chops (page 197)

WEEK 3 SHOPPING LIST

DAIRY			
blue cheese	low-fat shredded	1% or fat-free milk	smoked Cheddar or
eggs	Cheddar cheese	reduced-fat Mexican	Gouda cheese
fat-free plain yogurt	low-fat sour cream	blend cheese	soy milk

FRUITS AND VEGETABLES			
avocados	grape tomatoes	mushrooms	romaine lettuce
basil leaves	green and red bell	plum tomatoes	strawberries
blueberries	peppers	raspberries	sweet potatoes
cilantro	lettuce	red cabbage	tomatoes
flat-leaf parsley	limes	red onion	yellow onions
frozen corn kernels	mango		

BREADS, CEREALS, AND PASTAS			
Barilla Plus multigrain spaghetti	Kashi Honey Sunshine cereal	whole-wheat bread whole-wheat hamburger	whole-wheat pasta spirals
corn tortillas	old-fashioned rolled oats	buns	whole-wheat tortillas

BEANS, NUTS, AND RICE			
black beans	brown rice	red beans	

MEATS AND FISH			
bone-in pork chops	sliced deli turkey	1 pound ground turkey	medium to large frozen
1 or 2 packages chicken tenders	breast flank steak	lean ham steak mahimahi fillets	shrimp snapper or tilapia fillets

OTHER			
barbecue sauce	canned shrimp	fat-free mayonnaise	pickled ginger
blackening spices	canned tuna	maple syrup	Smart Balance Omega
canned crushed tomatoes	chicken stock cinnamon	Newman's Own balsamic vinaigrette	peanut butter wasabi paste
canned diced tomatoes with chile peppers	dry grill seasoning	oregano	whey protein powder

WEEK 4 SUGGESTED MEALS

BREAKFASTS	LUNCHES	DINNERS
Easy, Cheesy Breakfast Burrito (page 181)	Pesto Shrimp Pasta (page 203)	Peaches and Pork Chops (page 215)
Quick Thick Yogurt with Extras (page 179)	Turkey and cheese sandwich	Smoked Mozzarella Meatballs (page 214)
American-English Egg Sandwich (page 178)	Cold Hot Tuna Sandwich (page 188)	Spicy Sea Bass (page 208)
Protein Oatmeal Powerboost (page 180)	Pita Pizza (page 189)	Greek-Style Stuffed Chicken (page 207)
Kellogg's All-Bran extra fiber cereal	Greek Salad (page 188)	Grilled Sausage with The Works (page 209)

WEEK 4 SHOPPING LIST

DAIRY			
blue cheese	low-fat American cheese	low-fat Cheddar cheese	1% or fat-free milk
eggs	low-fat blueberry and	low-fat mozzarella	$^1/_2$ pound smoked
feta cheese	plain yogurt	cheese	mozzarella
Gorgonzola cheese			

FRUITS AND VEGETABLES			
apples	escarole or endive	peaches or nectarines	red onions
arugula	green beans	pineapple	romaine lettuce
avocado	lemon	portobello mushrooms	ruby red grapefruit
baby spinach	mixed greens	raspberries	shredded red cabbage
blueberries	onion	red and yellow bell	strawberries
cherry tomatoes	parsley	peppers	tomatoes

BREADS, CEREALS, AND PASTAS			
Kellogg's All-Bran Extra	orzo	Thomas' Oatmeal &	whole-wheat pasta
Fiber cereal	polenta	Honey english muffins	whole-wheat pitas
low-fat whole-grain	rolled oats	whole-wheat bread	whole-wheat tortillas
granola			

BEANS, NUTS, AND RICE		
almonds	pine nuts	walnuts

MEATS AND FISH			
Canadian bacon	lean ground beef	14 medium precooked	2 sea bass or cod fillets
chicken breasts	lean ham	shrimp	sliced deli turkey breast
chicken sausage		pork chops	

OTHER			
canned crushed tomatoes	honey	pesto	sun-dried tomatoes
canned tuna	marinara sauce	pickled ginger	whey protein powder
chopped olives	marinated artichoke		
fat-free mayonnaise	hearts		

BELLY OFF! CLUB REAL MEAL RECIPES

BREAKFASTS

American-English Egg Sandwich

2	large egg whites
1	large whole egg
1	teaspoon flaxseeds (whole)
1	whole-wheat English muffin, toasted
1	slice Canadian bacon
1	slice low-fat American cheese
1	teaspoon ketchup (optional)

1. Scramble the eggs in a bowl. Add the flaxseed to the mixture.

2. Cook in a nonstick skillet in a tiny bit of butter.

3. Put the eggs on a toasted English muffin. Top with bacon, cheese, and ketchup (if using).

MAKES ONE SERVING.

Per serving: 335 calories, 31 g protein, 31 g carbohydrates, 10 g fat (3 g saturated), 5 g fiber

Quick Thick Yogurt with Extras

1   cup fat-free or low-fat blueberry yogurt

1   handful of fresh or frozen blueberries

¼   cup slivered almonds

¼   cup low-fat whole-grain granola

1. Spoon yogurt into a bowl.

2. Stir in the blueberries, almonds, and granola.

MAKES ONE SERVING.

Per serving: 366 calories, 15 g protein, 42 g carbohydrates, 16 g fat
(1 g saturated), 6 g fiber

Huevos Rancheros Wrap

2   whole eggs

1   scallion, sliced

1   medium whole-wheat tortilla

2   tablespoons shredded reduced-fat Mexican blend cheese

1   tablespoon chopped cilantro

2   tablespoons salsa

1. Beat the eggs and scallion in a microwavable bowl.

2. Microwave the mixture for 2 minutes.

3. Spoon the eggs onto a tortilla, top with the cheese, cilantro, and salsa.

4. Roll up.

MAKES ONE SERVING.

Per serving: 270 calories, 20 g protein, 24 g carbohydrates, 3 g fat
(4.7 g saturated), 3 g fiber

SUPERSHOT
Spice Your Coffee

Sprinkle cinnamon on everything—toast, cereal, bananas, coffee, applesauce, yogurt, whatever. Studies show cinnamon improves insulin sensitivity so your body won't need as much of the hormone to keep your blood sugar in check.

Protein Oatmeal Powerboost

1   cup rolled oats

1   cup low-fat milk

½   cup fresh or frozen blueberries or strawberries

     Dash of salt

     Dash of ground cinnamon

     Sugar substitute or sugar to taste

1   scoop whey protein powder

1. Combine the oats and milk in a large microwavable bowl.

2. Microwave for 1 minute, stir, then microwave for another minute.

3. Mix in the berries, salt, cinnamon, and sugar substitute or sugar.

IMPORTANT: Let the oatmeal cool a bit before mixing in the protein powder. (Very hot oatmeal can cause protein powder to lump and sour.)

MAKES ONE SERVING.

Per serving: 585 calories, 43 g protein, 80 g carbohydrates, 11 g fat (3.6 g saturated), 10 g fiber

Easy, Cheesy Breakfast Burrito

½	cup diced lean ham
1	large whole-wheat tortilla
1	large whole egg, and 3 large egg whites, beaten
¼	cup shredded low-fat Cheddar or Swiss cheese
2	tablespoons salsa

1. In a nonstick skillet coated with cooking spray, sauté the diced ham over medium-high heat.

2. Place the cooked ham in the tortilla.

3. Add more cooking spray into the skillet and scramble the eggs together.

4. Add the cooked eggs to the tortilla and top with the cheese and salsa. Fold.

MAKES ONE SERVING.

Per serving: 419 calories, 43 g protein, 28 g carbohydrates, 14 g fat (4 g saturated), 2 g fiber

SUPERSHOT
Lick Salt

Choose Swiss cheese over Cheddar. Ounce for ounce, Cheddar has three times more sodium than Swiss.

Hill Country Omelet

⅓	cup chopped scallions
¼	cup diced onion
¼	cup canned chopped green chile peppers
¼	cup frozen corn kernels, thawed
½	cup chopped green or red bell pepper
	Pinch of ground cumin
4	egg whites
2	eggs
2	tablespoons fat-free milk
¼	teaspoon ground black pepper
	Pinch of salt
5½	ounces shredded low-fat Cheddar cheese
2	tablespoons medium-hot salsa (optional)

1. Coat a nonstick pan with cooking spray and heat over medium heat.

2. Add the scallions, onion, chile peppers, corn, and bell peppers.

3. Cook until the onions are translucent, then add the cumin and transfer to a small bowl.

4. Wipe out the skillet; coat with cooking spray.

5. In a bowl whisk together the egg whites, eggs, milk, black pepper, and salt. Pour half of the mixture into the skillet and cook, occasionally scraping the bottom of the pan, for 2 to 3 minutes. Sprinkle half of the Cheddar cheese and half of the vegetable mixture over the eggs. Cook, without stirring, for 3 to 4 minutes, or until the bottom is golden brown and the eggs are set. Using a spatula, flip the omelet in half and transfer to a plate. Top with half of the salsa (if using).

6. Coat the pan with cooking spray and repeat the procedure with the remaining ingredients for the second serving.

MAKES 2 SERVINGS.

Per serving: 288 calories, 34 g protein, 13.4 g carbohydrates, 10.7 g fat (5 g saturated), 3 g fiber

Chocolate Power Oatmeal

$1/2$ cup oat bran

$1/2$ cup oats

$1/3$ cup water

1   scoop chocolate whey protein powder

1. Microwave the oat bran, oats, and water for 3 to 4 minutes.

2. Let cool, then stir in the protein powder.

MAKES ONE SERVING.

Per serving: 333 calories, 25 g protein, 60 g carbohydrates, 6.8 g fat
(1 g saturated), 12 g fiber

FAT FACT

1,490

Calories in IHOP's
Big Steak Omelette.
You would need to
cross-country ski
10 miles to burn
that off.

Quick and Healthy Oatmeal

$1/2$ cup old-fashioned oats

1   cup soy milk or water

$1/4$ cup blueberries or raspberries

1   tablespoon maple syrup

1. Combine the oats and milk or water in a medium saucepan over
medium-high heat and bring to a boil. (Use more or less liquid to
reach desired consistency.)

2. Reduce heat and simmer for 5 minutes.

3. Serve topped with berries and maple syrup.

MAKES ONE SERVING.

Per serving: 373 calories, 18 g protein, 60 g carbohydrates, 8 g fat
(0.5 g saturated), 6 g fiber

LUNCHES

Mediterranean Wrap

1	large whole-wheat tortilla
2	tablespoons garlic-flavored hummus
¼	cup roasted red pepper strips
4	slices roast turkey breast
2	tablespoons chopped fresh mint leaves (optional)
¼	cup lettuce leaves

1. Lay the tortilla flat on a large cutting board. Spoon the hummus evenly over the tortilla to within ½ inch of edge. Lay the peppers evenly over the hummus. Layer on the turkey slices. Sprinkle with the mint (if using). Layer on the lettuce leaves.

2. Fold in the sides and then roll to form a wrap. Cut diagonally in half for that fancy deli look.

MAKES 2 WRAPS. Refrigerate, and you've got two lunches.

Per serving: 328 calories, 35.3 g protein, 31 g carbohydrates, 7 g fat (0.5 g saturated), 4.4 g fiber

Turkey-Avocado Cobb Salad

1	tablespoon water
2	tablespoons cider vinegar
1	teaspoon Dijon mustard
3	teaspoons olive oil
1	pound turkey breast cutlets
8	cups baby spinach
4	slices cooked turkey bacon, chopped
1	cup diced avocado
4	cherry tomatoes, halved
1	ounce blue cheese, crumbled
	Ground black pepper

FOR THE DRESSING:

Combine the water, vinegar, mustard, and 2 teaspoons of the olive oil in a bowl, and mix well.

FOR THE SALAD:

1. Preheat a grill pan on medium-high heat for 2 minutes.

2. Brush the turkey with the remaining olive oil and place in the grill pan.

3. Grill the turkey for 4 minutes, flip it, and continue cooking for about 3 minutes longer.

4. Remove the turkey from the heat. Let cool, then cut into chunks.

5. Dump the spinach and 2 tablespoons of the dressing into a large salad bowl, and toss to coat the leaves.

6. Arrange the turkey, turkey bacon, avocado, tomatoes, and cheese over the spinach so it looks nice, especially if you are serving someone else. (If it's only for you, just dump it on.)

7. Drizzle on the remaining dressing, and season with black pepper to taste.

MAKES 4 SERVINGS.

Per serving: 288 calories, 34 g protein, 10 g carbohydrates, 13.5 g fat
(3 g saturated), 5 g fiber

Eat-It-Cold Shrimp and Pasta Salad

$\frac{1}{2}$ cup whole-wheat fusilli pasta

1 can (3 ounces) shrimp, drained

$\frac{1}{2}$ cup grape tomatoes, halved

$\frac{1}{4}$ cup torn-up basil leaves (Don't have 'em?
Use spinach leaves.)

1 teaspoon Italian seasoning

1 teaspoon olive oil

1. In a medium pot of boiling water, cook the pasta 8 to 10 minutes. Drain in a colander and rinse with cold water until cool to the touch.

2. Place the pasta, shrimp, tomatoes, basil, Italian seasoning, and oil in a large bowl and toss to coat.

MAKES 2 SERVINGS. Make it for dinner, and take the rest for lunch tomorrow.

Per serving: 99 calories, 10 g protein, 10 g carbohydrates, 3 g fat
(0.5 g saturated), 2 g fiber

Belly Off! Pizza with The Works

1   whole-wheat pizza crust

¼   cup sun-dried tomato pesto

1   small zucchini, sliced

1   cup thinly sliced orange and yellow bell peppers

1   cup sliced fresh mushrooms

½   cup thinly sliced red onion

2   teaspoons olive oil

2   ounces fresh mozzarella cheese, thinly sliced

2   tablespoons grated Parmesan cheese

¾   cup sun-dried tomatoes

½   cup thinly sliced fresh basil leaves

1. Preheat the oven to 425°F. Place the crust on baking sheet.

2. Spread the crust with pesto.

3. Toss the zucchini, peppers, mushrooms, and onion with oil.

4. Place the vegetables in a medium skillet over medium-high heat and sauté in oil until vegetables are soft and excess liquid has evaporated, about 6 to 8 minutes.

5. Top the crust evenly with the cheeses. Arrange the vegetables over the cheese, and top with the sun-dried tomatoes. Bake 18 to 20 minutes, until the crust is baked through and crisp.

6. Sprinkle with the basil leaves. Let stand a few minutes before cutting into quarters.

NOTE: One serving is ¼ of the pie.

MAKES 4 SERVINGS.

Per serving: 301 calories, 16 g protein, 42 g carbohydrates, 11 g fat (3 g saturated), 7 g fiber

Greek Salad

3	cups torn romaine lettuce
1	cup torn escarole or curly endive
1/4	cup thinly sliced red onion
1/4	cup thinly sliced radishes
1	medium tomato, cut into 8 wedges
2	tablespoons lemon juice
2	teaspoons olive oil
1	tablespoon fat-free plain yogurt
1	teaspoon honey
1/4	teaspoon dried oregano
	Salt
	Ground black pepper

1. In a large salad bowl, combine the lettuce, escarole or endive, onion, radishes, and tomato wedges.

2. In a jar, combine the lemon juice, oil, yogurt, honey, and oregano; shake to mix. Add salt and pepper to taste. Pour over the salad. Toss well.

MAKES 4 SERVINGS.

Per serving: 48 calories, 1 g protein, 6 g carbohydrates, 2 g fat (0.4 g saturated), 2 g fiber

Cold Hot Tuna Sandwiches

1/4	cup fat-free mayonnaise
1/2	teaspoon wasabi paste
8	ounces canned tuna
8	slices whole-wheat bread
4	thin slices red onion
4	thin rings red bell pepper, seeded

1 cup sliced avocado

¼ cup sliced pickled ginger

lettuce leaves

1. In a small bowl, mix the mayonnaise and wasabi paste together.

2. Fork the tuna into the bowl, and combine with the mayo-wasabi mixture.

3. Spread an equal amount of the spicy tuna mixture on 4 slices of bread.

4. Top with an onion slice, pepper ring, avocado slice, 1 tablespoon of ginger, and a lettuce leaf, and the remaining slices of bread.

MAKES 4 SERVINGS.

Per serving: 308 calories, 22 g protein, 34 g carbohydrates, 9.5 g fat (1.7 g saturated), 7 g fiber

Pita Pizza

2 tablespoons marinara sauce

1 whole-wheat pita (6-inch diameter)

1 tablespoon Italian seasoning (or dried basil and oregano)

¼ cup diced pineapple

4 oz lean ham

½ cup shredded low-fat mozzarella cheese

1. Preheat the oven to 425°F.

2. Spread the marinara sauce over the pita, add the Italian seasoning, and top with the pineapple, ham, and cheese.

3. Bake the pita for 8 minutes on a baking sheet on the center oven rack.

MAKES 1 SERVING.

Per serving: 482 calories, 45 g protein, 36 g carbohydrates, 17 g fat (6.3 g saturated), 4 g fiber

SUPERSHOT
Go for the Green

Doctor your favorite
jarred pasta sauce
with ½ cup of frozen
chopped spinach,
which will add
vitamins and fiber.

Three-Alarm Sloppy Joes

2	cans (15 ounces each) barbecue baked beans
1	can (14 ounces) diced tomatoes
1½	tablespoons chili powder
1	tablespoon garlic powder
3	whole-wheat hamburger buns

1. Dump the beans, tomatoes (with juice), chili powder, and garlic powder into a large nonstick pan, cover and simmer for 10 minutes.

2. Slop an equal amount onto each bun.

MAKES 3 SERVINGS.

Per serving: 509 calories, 19 g protein, 90 g carbohydrates, 9.8 g fat (2.9 g saturated), 18.4 g fiber

DINNERS AND SIDES

One-Pot Chicken Pasta with a Kick

1	boneless, skinless chicken breast half
$1/2$	cup whole-wheat penne pasta
1	plum tomato, seeded and diced
2	tablespoons tomato paste
2	cloves garlic, minced
3	cups baby spinach
$1/4$	teaspoon red pepper flakes
	Coarse salt
1	tablespoon lemon juice

1. Chop the chicken into 1-inch chunks.

2. Boil salted water in a large pot, then cook the penne. (Follow directions on the box.) During the last 2 minutes of cooking, add the chicken chunks. Drain the pasta and chicken, but save $1/4$ cup of the water. Return the chicken and pasta to the original pot.

3. Add the diced tomato, tomato paste, garlic, spinach, and red pepper flakes.

4. Cook over medium heat, tossing until the spinach wilts. Season with salt. Remove from heat.

5. Stir in the reserved pasta water and lemon juice, which will create a light sauce.

MAKES 1 SERVING.

Per serving: 459 calories, 44 g protein, 63 g carbohydrates, 4 g fat (0.5 g saturated), 11 g fiber

IT WORKS FOR ME

"Try to eat dinner before 7 p.m. so your body has a chance to burn the calories before you go to bed. And learn to drink simply. Soda and juice are loaded with carbs. Learn to love water. If I crave sweet juice, I eat fruit instead."

—Andrew Lebson, Brooklyn, NY, who lost 100 pounds

Grilled Asparagus

1   bunch asparagus, thick ends removed

1   tablespoon extra-virgin olive oil

Coarse sea salt

Fresh cracked pepper

1. Place the asparagus on a plate and brush with the olive oil.

2. Using tongs, place the asparagus on a hot grill, and roast, turning often until lightly browned. (You can also roast it on a baking sheet in an oven preheated to 400°F. Toss frequently.)

3. Plate and sprinkle with coarse sea salt and a few cranks from a pepper mill.

MAKES 4 SERVINGS.

Per serving: 44.8 calories, 1.1 g protein, 2.2 g carbohydrates, 3.6 g fat (0.5 g saturated), 1.1 g fiber

Blue Plate Special Meatloaf

1/3	cup sun-dried tomatoes
1/2	teaspoon olive oil
1/3	cup chopped onions
1/2	cup chopped celery
1/2	cup chopped green bell peppers
2	cloves garlic, minced
1/2	teaspoon dried thyme
1/8	teaspoon ground black pepper
1	pound extra-lean ground beef
8	ounces ground turkey breast
1/3	cup low-carb ketchup
1/4	cup toasted bread crumbs
1/4	cup fat-free milk
1/4	cup fat-free egg substitute
2	teaspoons dried dill
2	teaspoons Worcestershire sauce

1. Preheat an oven to 350°F. Coat a 9" × 5" loaf pan with nonstick cooking spray.

2. Place the tomatoes in a small bowl. Cover with boiling water and let stand for 10 minutes or until the tomatoes are softened. Drain the tomatoes and chop. Set aside.

3. Warm the oil in a medium nonstick skillet over medium heat. Add the onions, celery, bell peppers, garlic, thyme, and black pepper. Cook, stirring occasionally, for 8 to 10 minutes.

4. In a large bowl, mix together the beef and turkey. Then add the ketchup, bread crumbs, milk, egg substitute, dill, Worcestershire sauce, tomatoes, and cooked vegetables. Mix well.

5. Press the mixture into the pan. Bake for 1 hour or until golden brown and no longer pink in the center when tested with a knife. Let stand for 10 minutes before slicing.

MAKES 6 SERVINGS.

Per serving: 192 calories, 27.3 g protein, 11.5 g carbohydrates, 5 g fat (1.6 g saturated), 1.3 g fiber

Taco Salad

1	pound lean ground beef
1	package taco seasoning, plus water as directed on package
8	cups shredded romaine lettuce
1	can (11 ounces) corn, drained
2	cups diced tomatoes
2	cups blue corn tortilla chips, broken up
1	bottle (18 ounces) low-fat Catalina salad dressing

1. Cook the ground beef in a large skillet over medium heat until browned. Drain the fat. Add the taco seasoning and water. Stir until the mixture begins to thicken. Remove from heat.

2. In a large bowl, combine the lettuce, corn, tomatoes, and dressing.

3. Top with the meat and chips just before serving.

MAKES 8 SERVINGS.

Per serving: 338 calories, 14.7 g protein, 39 g carbohydrates, 13 g fat (4 g saturated), 3.9 g fiber

Hot Smoked Oyster Dip

1   can (9 ounces) sour cream and onion dip

1   teaspoon Worcestershire sauce

¼   teaspoon hot sauce

1   tablespoon chopped fresh parsley

1   can (3.5 ounce) smoked oysters

1. Mix everything except the oysters in a microwavable bowl. Set aside.

2. Chop the oysters and stir them into the dip with their liquid.

3. Microwave on high for about $1\frac{1}{2}$ minutes, stopping to stir every 30 seconds.

4. Serve with pita triangles or reduced-fat Triscuits.

MAKES 10 SERVINGS.

Per serving: 65 calories, 3 g protein, 4 g carbohydrates, 5 g fat (3 g saturated), 1 g fiber

FIT FACT
Candy bars with almonds deliver almost twice the fiber content of bars without the healthful nuts.

BBQ Beer Ribs

$\frac{1}{2}$ can beer

$1\frac{1}{2}$ cups spicy tomato juice cocktail

1 cup honey barbecue sauce

8 boneless country-style pork ribs (6 ounces each), fat trimmed

1. Dump all the ingredients into a Ziploc bag. Stick the bag in the fridge for 2 hours or overnight to marinate.

2. Cook the ribs on a hot grill for 15 minutes, turning frequently.

MAKES 8 SERVINGS.

Per serving: 352 calories; 33 g protein, 5 g carbohydrates, 17 g fat (6 g saturated), 0 g fiber

Better-for-You Fries

2 large russet potatoes, sliced lengthwise into $\frac{1}{4}$-inch strips

1 egg white, lightly beaten

$\frac{1}{4}$ teaspoon paprika

Salt

Ground black pepper

1. Preheat the oven to 400°F. Coat a baking sheet with cooking spray.

2. Brush the potatoes with the egg white. Sprinkle with the paprika. Bake for about 20 minutes, or until the fries are nicely browned. Season with salt and pepper to taste.

MAKES 4 SERVINGS.

Per serving: 150 calories, 4.9 g protein, 32 g carbohydrates, 0.2 g fat, 3.5 g fiber

Maple Mustard Pork Chops

1   tablespoon maple syrup

1   tablespoon Dijon mustard

1   teaspoon olive oil

1   small clove garlic, crushed

     Salt and pepper to taste

2   bone-in pork chops

1. Preheat a cast-iron skillet to medium-high.

2. In a small bowl, stir together the syrup, mustard, oil, garlic, salt, and pepper.

3. Place the chops and mustard mixture inside a large Ziploc plastic bag, then shake thoroughly to coat the chops.

4. Place the chops on the skillet, cooking 3 to 4 minutes per side. In the last minute of cooking, pour the remaining mustard mixture onto the chops.

5. Eat with a microwaved sweet potato.

MAKES 2 SERVINGS.

Per serving (including sweet potato): 380 calories, 35 g protein, 36 g carbohydrates, 11 g fat (3 g saturated), 4 g fiber

Frank's Flank Steak

1½	pounds (approx.) flank steak
⅔	cup balsamic vinegar
1	tablespoon cracked black pepper
3	cloves garlic
¼	cup olive oil

1. Jab the steak with a big fork in several places to create holes for the marinade to seep in.

2. Mix all the marinade ingredients in a large Ziploc bag, reserving ¼ cup. Drop the steak into the bag, and shake to coat. Put the bag in the refrigerator for at least an hour. You can also allow it to marinate overnight.

3. Grill over medium heat for about 6 minutes per side for medium rare. Baste with the reserved marinade.

4. Slice the meat diagonally across the grain in thin slices and drizzle with the marinade.

MAKES 4 SERVINGS.

Per serving: 393 calories, 48 g protein, 8 g carbohydrates, 14 g fat (5.5 g saturated), 0 fiber

HAVE A COW
How to Choose the Leanest Cuts of Beef

You don't have to give up beef to get rid of your gut. Beef can be part of a healthy diet as long as you keep saturated fat and cholesterol to a minimum by choosing the leanest cuts of meat and paying attention to serving size. Keep servings to between 3 and 5 ounces. A 3-ounce serving of cooked lean beef will contain about 8.5 grams of total fat and 3.2 grams of saturated fat. Remember, beef shrinks during cooking. For a 3-ounce serving of cooked meat, start with 4 ounces of uncooked boneless meat. The leanest cuts of beef come from the loin and legs of the animal:

• Top round	• Tenderloin	• Sirloin
• Top loin	• Eye of round	• Round tip

Beef is graded according to fat marbling: prime, choice, and select. Select is the leanest grade. Buy lean cuts closely trimmed of fat, or trim them yourself at home before you cook. When using less tender cuts, such as round cuts, marinate to tenderize. It's the acidic vinegar, wine, or citrus juice in marinades that tenderizes the meat, not the oil. So you can reduce total fat and calories without losing the tenderizing effect by replacing the oil with water.

Pork 'n' Greens

1	pork tenderloin (1 pound)
½	bottle Lawry's 30-Minute Marinade Sesame Ginger with Mandarin Orange Juice
1	bag (6 ounces) fresh spinach
2	cups cooked brown rice

1. Put the tenderloin in a large Ziploc bag and dump in ½ bottle of the Sesame Ginger marinade. Stick in fridge for 30 minutes.

2. Preheat the oven to 375°F. (Pork tenderloin is also wonderful on the barbecue grill.)

3. Place the tenderloin in a rectangular baking dish. Brush the pork with marinade from the bag.

4. Bake the tenderloin, uncovered, for 40 to 45 minutes, until the pork is no longer pink in the center.

5. While the pork is cooking, put a half inch of water into a large pot, add a steaming grid, and steam the spinach.

6. After removing the pork from the oven, let the meat sit for 5 minutes before carving. Cut into 1-inch slices. Serve with the spinach and brown rice.

MAKES 2 SERVINGS.

Per serving: 567 calories, 55 g protein, 70 g carbohydrates, 6.7 g fat (1.9 g saturated), 8 g fiber

Spicy Chicken Kickoff "Wings"

FAT FACT
Breaded chicken
and fish may provide
you with a good
source of protein,
but they can also
contain high
amounts of
unhealthy fat.

3	teaspoons honey
3	tablespoons hot sauce
2	tablespoons low-sodium Worcestershire sauce
1/2	teaspoon minced garlic
1/2	teaspoon paprika
12	chicken tenders

1. Preheat a nonstick skillet on medium-high.

2. Stir together the honey, hot sauce, Worcestershire sauce, garlic, and paprika in a small bowl. Microwave for 10 seconds, stirring if the honey clumps.

3. Place the chicken and half of the spice mixture in a large Ziploc bag and shake until coated.

4. Pour the coated tenders into the skillet and cook for 1 to 2 minutes per side.

5. Toss with the remaining spice mixture to coat them. Eat with celery sticks, baby carrots, and 4 tablespoons (2 tablespoons per serving) of a good, chunky blue cheese dressing that's reasonably low in fat, such as Ken's Steak House Lite.

MAKES 2 SERVINGS.

Per serving (including sides): 466 calories, 33 g protein, 54 g carbohydrates, 14 g fat (5 g saturated), 5 g fiber

Tuscan-Style Chicken Pasta

2	ounces Barilla Plus multigrain penne pasta
2	chicken breasts, 4 to 5 ounces each, pounded to an even 1/4-inch thickness
1	teaspoon olive oil
4	cups baby spinach leaves
1	cup cannellini beans, rinsed
1	clove garlic, crushed
1/2	teaspoon dried rosemary, finely chopped
2	heaping tablespoons diced roasted red bell pepper
2	tablespoons grated Parmesan
	Salt and pepper to taste

1. Boil 1 1/2 quarts of water, drop in the penne, stir, and cook until the pasta is al dente (about 9 to 11 minutes).

2. While the pasta cooks, sear the chicken in a skillet, to which you've added the olive oil, on medium-high (about 4 to 5 minutes per side), seasoning each side with a pinch of salt and pepper as the other side cooks. Remove the chicken from the skillet and set it aside.

3. Reduce skillet heat to medium. Add the spinach, beans, garlic, rosemary, and bell peppers. Turn frequently until the spinach wilts (about 1 to 2 minutes).

4. Slice the chicken and toss it with drained pasta and the spinach-and-bean mixture. Top each serving with 1 tablespoon of the cheese.

MAKES 2 SERVINGS.

Per serving: 430 calories, 40 g protein, 45 g carbohydrates, 8 g fat
(2 g saturated), 7 g fiber

Cheese 'n' Chili Chicken

1½	tablespoons of your favorite dry grill seasoning
1	pound chicken breast tenders
2½	cups drained red chili beans
1	can (8 ounces) diced tomatoes with chile peppers
¼	cup barbecue sauce
⅓	cup chicken stock
¼	cup grated smoked Cheddar or Gouda cheese

1. Smear the grill seasoning over the chicken tenders, then sear them in a medium-hot nonstick skillet that you've coated with cooking spray. Cook for about 2 minutes per side.

2. Reduce the heat to low and add the beans, tomatoes, barbecue sauce, and stock. Stir well to blend.

3. Let the mixture simmer for 10 minutes, stirring occasionally. When you're ready to serve, top it with the cheese.

MAKES 4 SERVINGS.

Per serving: 315 calories, 37 g protein, 35 g carbohydrates, 3.7 g fat (1.7 g saturated), 9 g fiber

Pesto Shrimp Pasta

4	ounces Barilla Plus penne pasta
12–14	medium-size precooked, peeled shrimp
3	cups chopped baby spinach
1	tomato, chopped
3	tablespoons ready-made pesto
3	tablespoons crumbled Gorgonzola cheese
2	tablespoons diced walnuts

1. Boil the pasta according to the package directions. If you're using frozen shrimp, defrost them by running warm water over them.

2. Drain the pasta. Transfer the pasta to a large bowl and add the spinach, tomato, pesto, cheese, and walnuts, stirring well to help wilt the spinach and mix in the pesto.

3. Eat with mixed greens and 2 or 3 slices of raw tomato, sprinkled lightly with salt and drizzled with balsamic vinaigrette.

MAKES 2 SERVINGS.

Per serving (including salad): 490 calories, 27 g protein, 47 g carbohydrates, 22 g fat (6 g saturated), 8 g fiber

FIT FACT

50

Percent reduction in your risk of developing a degenerative eye disease if you eat oily fish containing DHA omega-3 fatty acid at least once a week

Blackened Snapper with Mango Salsa

1	mango (skin and seed removed), cut into cubes
1	ripe avocado (skin and pit removed), cut into cubes
	Juice of 1 lime
¼	cup minced onion
½	cup chopped cilantro
	Salt and pepper
2	snapper, catfish, or tilapia fillets, 4 to 5 ounces each
1	tablespoon blackening spices
1	tablespoon vegetable oil

1. Combine the mango, avocado, lime juice, onion, and cilantro in a mixing bowl. Season with salt and pepper.

2. Preheat a large sauté or grill pan over high heat and add enough oil to coat it.

3. Rub the fillets with enough of the blackening spice to thoroughly cover each side. When the oil is hot (almost smoking), carefully add the fillets to the pan and cook for 2 to 3 minutes per side, until a nice, dark crust has developed. The fish is done when it flakes easily with light pressure from your finger.

4. Top each fillet with the mango salsa.

5. Eat with brown rice and black beans.

MAKES 2 SERVINGS.

Per serving (with rice and beans): 430 calories, 40 g protein, 45 g carbohydrates, 8 g fat (2 g saturated), 7 g fiber

Shrimp Fra Diavolo

2	teaspoons red pepper flakes
1/2	tablespoon extra-virgin olive oil
1	medium yellow onion, chopped
2	cloves garlic, minced
1/4	teaspoon dried oregano or thyme
14	ounces crushed tomatoes
4	ounces dried whole-wheat spaghetti
12	ounces shrimp, peeled and deveined
	Salt and pepper to taste
2	tablespoons chopped flat-leaf parsley

1. Boil a large pot of salted water for the pasta.

2. Heat a large sauté pan over medium heat. Add the red pepper flakes, oil, onion, garlic, and oregano or thyme, and cook until the onions are soft. Add the tomatoes.

3. Drop the pasta into the boiling water and cook according to the package directions.

4. Add the shrimp to the sauce and season with salt and pepper. Cook for 3 to 4 minutes. Drain the pasta, toss with as much of the sauce as you like, and garnish with parsley.

5. Eat with a simple green salad tossed with olive oil and balsamic vinegar.

MAKES 2 SERVINGS.

Per serving: 519 calories, 46.4 g protein, 66 g carbohydrates, 8 g fat (1.4 g saturated), 7.4 g fiber

FIT FACT
1 slice of whole-wheat toast with 2 slices of avocado, tomato, sea salt, and cracked black pepper is one heck of a mid-afternoon snack.

Chipotle Turkey Burgers

8	ounces lean ground turkey
1/4	teaspoon salt
1/4	teaspoon pepper
	Pinch of cumin
1/2	avocado, sliced
1	tomato, sliced
1/2	red onion, thinly sliced
2	wheat or whole-grain buns, toasted
2	tablespoons low-fat sour cream
2	tablespoons chipotle salsa

1. Mix the meat, salt, pepper, and cumin, and form it into two equal patties.

2. Preheat a skillet or frying pan over medium-high heat. Coat with a bit of oil and add the burgers, cooking them for 4 to 5 minutes per side, until slightly firm to the touch.

3. Dress each bun with avocado slices, tomato, and red onion. Top with the burger, sour cream, and salsa.

MAKES 2 SERVINGS.

Per serving: 419 calories, 27 g protein, 37 g carbohydrates, 21 g fat (5 g saturated), 7 g fiber

Greek-Style Stuffed Chicken

2   tablespoons chopped sun-dried tomatoes

2   tablespoons crumbled feta cheese

2   tablespoons chopped olives

1   teaspoon minced garlic

1   tablespoon pine nuts

1   tablespoon balsamic vinegar

2   chicken breasts (5 to 6 ounces each)

    Extra-virgin olive oil

    Salt and pepper

1. Preheat the oven to 450°F. Toss together the tomatoes, feta cheese, olives, garlic, pine nuts, and vinegar.

2. Rub the chicken with olive oil, salt, and pepper. Using a small, sharp knife, carefully cut a slit along the thick part of each chicken breast, creating a pocket. Add enough stuffing to fill each pocket and transfer the chicken to a baking sheet.

3. Bake for 15 minutes. Top with any remaining stuffing.

4. Eat with 1 cup cooked orzo mixed with sautéed spinach.

MAKES 2 SERVINGS.

Per serving (including sides): 680 calories, 65 g protein, 51 g carbohydrates, 23 g fat (5 g saturated), 4 g fiber

Spicy Sea Bass

1/2	tablespoon olive oil
2	fillets, 6-ounces each of sea bass, cod, or other firm white fish
1/2	cup white wine
1	small onion, sliced
1/2	cup pitted, chopped green olives
1	can (12 ounces) whole peeled tomatoes
2	cloves garlic, minced
1	teaspoon crushed red pepper
	Salt and pepper

1. Heat a large sauté pan over medium-high heat. Add the olive oil.

2. Season the fish with salt and pepper. When the oil is hot, add the fillets flesh side down and cook for 3 minutes, until a crust has formed. Remove the fish from the pan and set aside.

3. Add the wine and onion to the pan and cook for 3 minutes. Add the olives, tomatoes, garlic, and red pepper and cook for another 3 minutes. Season with salt and pepper.

4. Return the fish to the pan. Baste the fillets with the simmering tomato sauce. Cook until the flesh flakes with gentle pressure from your finger (5 to 7 minutes).

MAKES 2 SERVINGS.

Per serving: 400 calories, 35 g protein, 13 g carbohydrates, 19 g fat (2 g saturated), 2 g fiber

Grilled Sausage with The Works

$\frac{1}{2}$ tablespoon extra-virgin olive oil

2 links precooked chicken sausage (Try feta cheese or sun-dried tomato varieties.)

1 red or yellow bell pepper, sliced

1 medium red onion, sliced

1 large portobello mushroom cap, sliced

2 cloves garlic, minced

$\frac{1}{2}$ teaspoon red pepper flakes

1 tablespoon balsamic vinegar

Salt and pepper to taste

"Avoid taking extra bites of leftover food when you are cleaning up after dinner—especially an Italian dinner; they can add up to hundreds of extra calories a day. Suck on a sugar-free lollipop if you must to avoid becoming a human vacuum cleaner."

—Anthony Piazza,
Staten Island, NY,
who lost 12 pounds

1. Heat a grill pan or cast-iron skillet over medium-high heat and add the olive oil.

2. When the oil begins to smoke, add the sausage, pepper, onion, and mushroom. Cook for 3 to 4 minutes, moving the vegetables with a pair of tongs or a spatula so they cook evenly. Add the garlic, pepper flakes, and vinegar and cook for another 3 to 4 minutes, until the vegetables and sausage are browned and the vinegar has been absorbed.

3. Season with salt and pepper and serve with $\frac{1}{2}$ cup soft polenta, prepared according to the package directions.

MAKES 2 SERVINGS.

Per serving: 460 calories, 28 g protein, 51 g carbohydrates, 16 g fat (8 g saturated), 7 g fiber

Mediterranean-Style Cod

1	pint cherry tomatoes
$\frac{1}{2}$	bulb fennel or yellow onion, sliced thin
$\frac{1}{2}$	tablespoon extra-virgin olive oil
	Salt and pepper to taste
2	tablespoons prepared olive tapenade
2	cod, halibut, or snapper fillets, 6 ounces each

1. Preheat oven to 400°F.

2. Lay the tomatoes and fennel on a baking dish, and toss with the olive oil, salt, and pepper. Slather 1 tablespoon of the tapenade on each fish fillet and lay the fillets in the baking dish with the vegetables. Place the dish in the oven.

3. Roast for 10 to 12 minutes, until the tomatoes are soft and the flesh of the fish flakes with gentle pressure from your finger.

4. Serve each fillet with $\frac{1}{2}$ cup prepared couscous mixed with 2 tablespoons toasted pine nuts and chopped fresh basil.

MAKES 2 SERVINGS.

Per serving: 370 calories, 44 g protein, 21 g carbohydrates, 12 g fat (1.5 g saturated), 5 g fiber

Jerk Pork Kebabs and Sweet Potato Fries

FOR THE KEBABS

1   pork tenderloin (12 ounces), cut into 1-inch cubes

2   cups fresh pineapple or mango chunks

1   red bell pepper, cut into 1-inch pieces

1   large onion, cut into 1-inch slices

½   cup of prepared jerk sauce (try Busha Browne's Spicy Jerk Sauce or Walkerswood Jamaican Jerk Seasoning)

4   wooden skewers, presoaked in cold water for 30 minutes

FOR THE SWEET POTATO FRIES

1   large sweet potato

Olive oil

Salt

Chili powder

1. Preheat a grill or grill pan over high heat.

2. Assemble the kebabs by skewering pieces of pork, pineapple or mango, pepper, and onion, alternating as you go. Brush with half of the jerk sauce and place on the hot grill. Grill for 4 minutes a side, basting with the rest of the jerk sauce. The kebabs are done when the vegetables are lightly charred and the pork is firm to the touch.

3. Serve with sweet potato fries: Cut one large sweet potato into wedges, toss with olive oil, salt, and chili powder, and bake in a 450°F oven for 20 minutes.

MAKES 2 SERVINGS.

Per serving (including fries): 560 calories, 52 g protein, 52 g carbohydrates, 9 g fat (3 g saturated), 8 g fiber

IT WORKS FOR ME

"Cut simple carbs first. I stalled my progress by going for all the nonfat foods. Your body learns that if it's not going to get any fat, it's not going to give up any."

—David Vandelinde,
Elburn, IL,
who lost 175 pounds

Grilled Spicy Fish Tacos

    Canola oil

12   ounces mahi-mahi

1/2 tablespoon blackening spice

4   corn tortillas

1   mango, peeled, pitted, and cubed

1   avocado, peeled, pitted, and cubed

1/2 medium red onion, diced

1   handful cilantro, chopped

2   limes

1   cup finely shredded red cabbage

    Salt and pepper

1/2 cup black beans

    Cumin

1. Clean and oil a grill or grill pan thoroughly. Preheat to medium-high.

2. Drizzle a light coating of oil over the fish, and rub on the blackening spice. Place the fish on the grill and cook, undisturbed, for 4 minutes. Carefully flip with a spatula and cook for another 4 minutes. Remove. Before turning off the grill, warm the tortillas directly on the surface for 1 to 2 minutes.

3. Make the mango salsa by combining the mango, avocado, red onion, cilantro, and the juice of one lime. Season to taste with salt and pepper.

4. Divide the fish evenly among the warm tortillas, add a bit of cabbage, and spoon the salsa on top. Serve each taco with a wedge of lime and 1/2 cup of black beans spiked with cumin.

MAKES 2 SERVINGS.

Per serving: 610 calories, 45 g protein, 75 g carbohydrates, 18 g fat (3 g saturated), 20 g fiber

Cedar-Plank Salmon

1   large, untreated cedar plank (Soak the cedar plank in
    water for at least 2 hours.)

1   large English cucumber, seeded and sliced

2   tablespoons rice-wine vinegar

1   teaspoon red pepper flakes

2   teaspoons sesame seeds

2   tablespoons fresh mint or cilantro, chopped

2   salmon fillets, 6 ounces each

    Salt and pepper

1. Combine the cucumbers, rice-wine vinegar, red pepper flakes, sesame seeds, and herbs in a mixing bowl. Season to taste with salt and pepper.

2. Preheat the grill on high. Lay the cedar plank on the grill. Season the salmon with salt and pepper. When the plank begins to smoke, lay the fillets on it, skin side down. Close the top, and grill for 10 to 12 minutes, until the salmon flakes with light pressure from your finger.

3. Top the salmon with the cucumbers, and garnish with a sprinkling of sesame seeds.

MAKES 2 SERVINGS.

Per serving: 300 calories, 36 g protein, 8 g carbohydrates, 12 g fat (1.5 g saturated), 2 g fiber

Smoked Mozzarella Meatballs

12	ounces lean ground beef
1	slice bread, torn into tiny pieces and soaked in milk
2	eggs
1/2	cup chopped fresh parsley, plus more for garnish
1	onion, chopped
4	cloves garlic, minced
	Salt and pepper
1/2	pound smoked mozzarella, cut into 1/2-inch cubes
1	tablespoon olive oil
1	can (32 ounces) crushed tomatoes

1. Mix the beef with the bread, eggs, 1/2 cup parsley, half the onion and garlic, and a generous sprinkling of salt and pepper. Without overworking the meat, form meatballs.

2. Hold each meatball in the palm of one hand and use the thumb of your other hand to make an indentation in the meatball. Drop in a cheese cube, and then carefully fold the meat back over to cover.

3. Heat the oil in a large skillet or pot over medium heat and sear each meatball until brown all over. Remove to a plate. Pour off all but a little fat and add the remaining onion and garlic; sauté until light brown. Return the meatballs to the pan, add the tomatoes, and cook over low heat for 20 minutes to 1 hour.

4. Season the sauce with salt and pepper. Serve over whole-wheat pasta and garnish with parsley.

MAKES 4 SERVINGS.

Per serving: 460 calories, 41 g protein, 26 g carbohydrates, 22 g fat (11 g saturated), 6 g fiber

Peaches and Pork Chops

2	bone-in pork chops, 8 ounces each, 1 inch thick
	Olive oil
	Salt and pepper
2	firm peaches or nectarines, halved and pitted
2	tablespoons pine nuts, toasted
1	small red onion, thinly sliced
½	cup crumbled blue cheese
1	tablespoon balsamic vinegar

1. Preheat a grill on high. Brush the pork with olive oil and season with salt and pepper. Grill for 4 to 5 minutes on each side.

2. While the chops cook, brush the peach halves with oil and add to the grill, facedown. Grill for 5 minutes or until soft. Remove, slice, and toss with the pine nuts, onion, blue cheese, and vinegar. Add salt and pepper to taste. Top each chop with half the salad and serve.

3. Eat with fresh arugula tossed with olive oil and lemon.

MAKES 2 SERVINGS.

Per serving: 430 calories, 38 g protein, 16 g carbohydrates, 24 g fat (9 g saturated), 2 g fiber

THE WORLD'S MOST NUTRITIOUS SALAD
How to Make a Meal Out of Rabbit Food

I love salad. Mostly because it involves demolition. You chop and dice vegetables with a chef's knife and tear hunks of crisp lettuce with your bare hands; and no matter how uncoordinated you are, you just can't screw it up. If you can make a mess, you can make a salad. Dump it all into a big bowl, sprinkle on some dressing, toss, and you've got a meal.

A meal, from salad? That's right. A real meal. The ultimate meal. If you add some protein and the right combination of vegetables, you can turn a little tossed salad into a satisfying muscle-building powerhouse of essential vitamins and antioxidants. Here's how to construct the world's most nutritious salad. Eat this and you won't need that horse pill of a multivitamin.

SPINACH

One cup of spinach gives you 58 micrograms (mcg) of folate. According to a study in the journal *Stroke* (Yeah, believe it or not, there's a magazine called *Stroke*.), consuming at least 300 mcg of folate a day reduces your risk of having a stroke by 20 percent and decreases your risk of developing heart disease by 13 percent. Other studies have found that folate helps protect against both Alzheimer's and cancer.

Essential Nutrients: Folate, fiber, protein, vitamin A, vitamin B_6, vitamin C, vitamin E, vitamin K, calcium, and potassium

Disease-Fighting Power: Heart disease, cancer, Alzheimer's, osteoporosis, diabetes, weight gain, hypertension, and depression

BROCCOLI

You get 294 milligrams (mg) of potassium in just three spears. According to Mayo Clinic researchers, potassium counteracts the effects of sodium by dilating blood vessels and increasing the amount of sodium excreted in your urine, thus lowering blood pressure and protecting against stroke.

Essential Nutrients: Potassium, calcium, fiber, vitamin A, vitamin B_6, vitamin C, vitamin K, folate, and lutein and zeaxanthin

Disease-Fighting Power: Heart disease, hypertension, cancer, osteoporosis, macular degeneration, Alzheimer's, diabetes, and weight gain

RED KIDNEY BEANS

A quarter cup of red kidney beans gives you 6,630 disease-fighting antioxidants, plus a full 3 grams of fiber. According to the American Dietetic Association, dietary fiber lowers blood cholesterol levels and helps normalize blood glucose and insulin levels, decreasing the risk of cardiovascular disease, metabolic syndrome, and type 2 diabetes.

Essential Nutrients: Protein, folate, antioxidants, fiber

Disease-Fighting Power: Heart disease, diabetes, cancer, and Alzheimer's

YELLOW BELL PEPPERS

Four strips of a yellow bell pepper provide 48 mg of free-radical-fighting vitamin C. (Free radicals are rogue molecules that can damage cells and lead to cancer.) According to a study in the *Journal of the American College of Nutrition*, levels of C-reactive protein—a blood marker for inflammation linked to heart disease—can be decreased by 24 percent if you consume 500 mg of vitamin C a day.

Plus, nutrition researchers from Arizona State University reported that vitamin C can help with weight loss by assisting in fat oxidation, or the body's ability to burn fat.

Essential Nutrients: Vitamin C, vitamin A, vitamin B_6, folate, and potassium

Disease-Fighting Power: Heart disease, cancer, Alzheimer's, weight gain, and hypertension

SWISS CHEESE

Four cubes of Swiss cheese provide 476 mg of calcium and 26 IU of vitamin D. In a 20-year study, British researchers determined that men who consume more than 190 mg of calcium and 67 IU of vitamin D a day have half the risk of stroke of men who consume less. Vitamin D has also been associated with a decrease in the risk of pancreatic, prostate, and testicular cancers. A study in the *Journal of the National Cancer Institute* found that men with higher blood levels of vitamin D had a 17 percent reduction in total cancer incidence and a 29 percent reduction in total cancer deaths.

Essential Nutrients: Calcium, vitamin D, protein, and vitamin B_{12}

Disease-Fighting Power: Osteoporosis, Alzheimer's, cancer, and stroke

CARROTS

Carrots are one of the richest sources of pro–vitamin A carotenoids, plant compounds that provide color and function as antioxidants. Just $1/4$ cup of shredded carrots provides 2,279 mcg of beta-carotene and 4,623 IU of vitamin A. According to a study in the journal *Thorax,* beta-carotene can slow the age-related decline of lung power. Vitamin A has also been shown to improve vision, bone growth, and cell division; help regulate the immune system; and decrease the risk of lung cancer.

Essential Nutrients: Vitamin A, vitamin C, vitamin K, fiber, and potassium

Disease-Fighting Power: Cancer, osteoporosis, weight gain, and hypertension

EXTRA-VIRGIN OLIVE OIL AND BALSAMIC VINEGAR

One tablespoon of olive oil delivers 10 grams of monounsaturated fat. Research shows that men with diets high in monounsaturated fat have higher testosterone levels than those who don't. Antioxidant-rich balsamic vinegar can improve vascular function when ingested with a high-fat food like olive oil, which contributes to a reduction in the risk of heart disease.

Essential Nutrients: Monounsaturated fat and antioxidants

Disease-Fighting Power: Adding olive oil to red, green, orange, or yellow fruits and vegetables increases the amount of heart-saving, cancer-fighting, vision-boosting, immune-repairing, bone-strengthening vitamins such as A, E, and K, as well as carotenoids.

SUNFLOWER SEEDS AND FLAXSEEDS

One tablespoon of sunflower seeds provides 8.35 mcg of selenium. Harvard researchers discovered that men with high levels of selenium have a 49 percent lower incidence of advanced prostate cancer than those with the lowest levels. One tablespoon of flaxseeds will give you 2.3 grams of omega-3 fatty acids, which are linked to reduced risk of heart disease, Alzheimer's, and depression. They have also been shown to inhibit cancer-cell growth.

Essential Nutrients: Selenium, vitamin E, and fiber

Disease-Fighting Power: Heart disease, cancer, Alzheimer's, depression, and diabetes

(continued)

THE WORLD'S MOST NUTRITIOUS SALAD—CONTINUED

ALMONDS

One tablespoon of almonds provides 2.2 grams of alpha-tocopherol, a type of vitamin E, which reduces the risk of Alzheimer's, according to a National Institute on Aging study. Another study showed that people who were clinically depressed had lower levels of alpha-tocopherol than their happy peers. Vitamin E also fights free-radical damage.

Essential Nutrients: Alpha-tocopherol, monounsaturated fat, protein, and fiber

Disease-Fighting Power: Alzheimer's, depression, cancer, heart disease, and diabetes

TOMATOES

Four cherry tomatoes will give you 1,748 mcg of lycopene. A study in the *Journal of the National Cancer Institute* found that increasing dietary lycopene intake to 30 mg reduces oxidative DNA damage to prostate tissues and decreases PSA levels.

Essential Nutrients: Lycopene, vitamin A, vitamin C, vitamin K, fiber, and potassium

Disease-Fighting Power: Cancer, heart disease, osteoporosis, diabetes, and hypertension

CHUNK LIGHT TUNA

Tuna, one of the best sources of protein, contains no trans fat, and a 3-ounce serving of chunk light contains 11 mg of heart-healthy niacin, which has been shown to help lower cholesterol and help your body process fat. University of Rochester researchers determined that niacin raises HDL cholesterol (the good kind) and lowers triglycerides more than most statins alone.

Essential Nutrients: Omega-3 fatty acids, niacin, protein, selenium, and vitamin B_{12}

Disease-Fighting Power: Heart disease and diabetes

RED-LEAF LETTUCE

Four leaves of red-leaf lettuce contain 1,213 mcg of antioxidants, 96 mcg of vitamin K (which has been shown to maintain bone mass), and 1,172 mcg of the carotenoids lutein and zeaxanthin. The National Institutes of Health found that lutein and zeaxanthin can decrease your risk of developing macular degeneration by 43 percent.

Essential Nutrients: Antioxidants, vitamin K, vitamin A, vitamin B_6, vitamin C, folate, and potassium

Disease-Fighting Power: Osteoporosis, macular degeneration, cancer, heart disease, hypertension, Alzheimer's, and weight gain

THE BELLY OFF! DIET WORLD'S MOST NUTRITIOUS SALAD

NUTRITION FACTS
CALORIES: 618
PROTEIN: 41 grams
CARBOHYDRATES: 35 grams
FAT: 37 grams (6 grams saturated)
FIBER: 14 grams
TRANS FAT: 0 grams
SODIUM: 178 milligrams

8

BELLY OFF! SUPERFOODS

Eat More Good Things

YOUR REFRIGERATOR is to losing weight as your tackle box is to catching fish.

Let me explain: If you're out on the lake and the walleye happen to be feeding on fathead minnows, but you don't have a lure resembling a fathead minnow in your tackle box, you're probably not going to catch any walleye. Likewise, if you're hungry but the only stuff in your fridge is fish sticks, Häagen-Dazs, and a six-pack of St. Pauli Girl, you're not going to advance your weight-loss efforts. A well-stocked refrigerator is like a well-appointed tackle box. It prepares you with options. And having lots of smart food options is essential in the quest to flatten your belly.

For most of our lives, we could blame bad food choices on the people who fed us: Mom, that cafeteria lady with the net on her head, Colonel Sanders, Ronald McDonald, Wendy, and Long John Silver. Not any

FIT FACT

14

Average number of years you add to your life if you eat lots of fruits and vegetables, don't smoke, exercise regularly, and drink in moderation, compared to people who don't follow these habits

more. We're adults now and free to make intelligent selections. Free to put whatever we want in that fridge.

The problem here is that there's something attached to us that influences our food choices: a tongue. A tongue that's covered in taste buds. Therefore, we tend to eat that which tastes good, even though it might not be very good for us. The tongue, as you may have heard, is one of the most powerful muscles in the body. But there's one that's stronger: your brain. If you fill it with knowledge of good, healthful foods, and listen to it, you can overpower that lustful tongue.

Below you'll find a listing of some of the most healthful foods to be had. These superfoods fight fat, stoke metabolism (your body's fat-burning furnace), deliver optimum energy, boost your immune system, and ward off the ravages of aging and disease. A wise bearded man once taught me that eating is an adventure in discipline and discernment. Get to know good food. Let your adventure begin here.

ARUGULA

Nothing against the venerable head of iceberg lettuce, but there are other foundations on which to build a nutritious salad. Peppery-flavored arugula is one of them; it contains about twice as much bone-building calcium and magnesium as iceberg. Other ways to extend your leafy green repertoire: romaine, red leaf, and green leaf lettuces; spinach; watercress; endive; red chard; and radicchio. For an easy path into unfamiliar salad-green territory, buy a package of spring mix, which contains many of the above.

ASPARAGUS

Asparagus is an excellent source of blood-building folate, a nutrient that is also important for mental function. In addition, it is one of the richest sources of rutin, a compound that strengthens capillary walls. And a 5.3-ounce serving delivers 3 grams of dietary fiber. If you haven't tried grilled asparagus yet, you're missing a real treat. Brush some olive oil over the stalks after snapping off the tough ends, and roast the asparagus on a hot grill for about 5 minutes, turning often to avoid charring. Top with cracked black pepper and sea salt.

AVOCADO

This is a good tool for weight loss because it's high in monounsaturated fats, which speed up your basal metabolic rate, while also delivering a quick feeling of fullness to help you avoid overeating. A study found that the increase in fat-burning ability prompted by monounsaturated fats was greatest for men who had a high waist-to-hip ratio, so the more belly you have to lose, the more fat this fatty acid will help to burn. Avocados are also high in beta-sitosterol, a compound that has been shown to lower cholesterol. And the folate (½ cup delivers about 25 percent of your daily value) and vitamin E in avocados may be protective against stroke.

BARILLA PLUS MULTIGRAIN SPAGHETTI

A far better choice than regular pasta, this spaghetti is based on a flour made from lentils, chickpeas, barley, flaxseed, wheat, and oat fiber. A 100-gram serving (about 1 cup) provides 17 grams of protein, 7 grams of dietary fiber, and 28 percent of your daily value of omega-3 fats.

BEANS AND LEGUMES

One of the healthiest sources of slow-burning carbohydrates, dietary fiber, and protein, beans and legumes are worthy of a spot on your daily menu. Variety makes that possible. Here's what the individual varieties offer:

Black beans: Rich in antioxidants called anthocyanins, which fight heart disease and cancer.

SUPERSHOT
Tuna Helper

If you don't like the fishy smell of fish, but want to ease yourself into eating more of this healthy protein, try a white fish such as striped bass, snapper, or halibut. Their neutral flavor and scent can convert those who are turned off by oilier fish such as tuna and salmon.

Garbanzo beans (chickpeas): In one study, a chick-pea-fortified diet slashed LDL ("bad") cholesterol levels by almost 5 percent. Toss them into salads.

Kidney beans: Rich in thiamin (vitamin B$_1$), which protects memory and brain function. Thiamin deficiency has been linked to Alzheimer's disease. Use in chili. Dump in spaghetti sauce.

Navy beans: Contain potassium, which regulates blood pressure and normal heart contractions.

Pinto beans: Rich in fiber, which helps stabilize blood sugar, lowering the risk of type 2 diabetes.

BEEF

Of course it's a prime source of protein, but it's also rich in two key muscle-building nutrients: iron and zinc. Plus, it's a great food source of creatine, your body's energy supply for pumping iron. Choose "rounds" or "loins"—butcherspeak for the leaner cuts. Another bonus from beef: selenium, a nutrient that may protect you from prostate cancer. Stanford University researchers found that men with low blood levels of this mineral are as much as five times more likely to develop prostate cancer than those with normal levels.

FAT FACT

Granola bars and energy bars are convenient for snacks but most are loaded with sugar, many with 24 grams or more. Read labels and choose those that have 24 grams of total carbohydrates or less. Some Atkins Advantage bars contain as little as 17 grams of carbs, but check the label—some flavors run considerably higher.

BEETS

This crimson vegetable is a powerhouse of folate and betaine. These two nutrients work in tandem to lower your blood levels of homocysteine, an inflammatory compound that can damage your arteries and increase your risk of heart disease. You'll reap more antioxidant benefits by eating raw fresh beets rather than their jarred cousins. Grate them into a salad.

BELL PEPPERS

Red, green, yellow, and orange—all are good sources of vitamin C, vitamin B$_6$, and folate. They contain lots of phytochemicals that can protect you from heart disease, cancer, stroke, and even cataracts.

BERRIES

Blueberries: Try to get ½ cup of these babies a day. Frozen ones are just as nutritious as fresh. Blueberries are packed with antioxidants and flavonoids, and contain some potassium. One particular antioxidant, pterostilbene, which is similar to the resveratrol in grapes, can stimulate liver cells to better break down fat and cholesterol, according to USDA scientists. Blueberries also fight inflammation, the key driver of many chronic diseases. Tip: The darker the berry, the more good stuff it contains.

Cranberries: Cranberries get the silver medal for having more antioxidants than all other common fruits, except for wild blueberries. Cranberries also can be called a natural probiotic, enhancing good bacteria levels in the gut.

Strawberries, raspberries, blackberries: All contain ellagic acid and a large number of polyphenols, which inhibit tumor growth. Raspberries and blackberries are loaded with fiber; you get 8 grams in just 1 cup. Strawberries deliver 3 per cup.

BLACK TEA

If you prefer this over green tea, go for it. Black tea offers all the antioxidant power of green tea with one exception: no EGCG, the cholesterol-lowering super catechin. Steep a bunch of tea bags to brew a big batch that'll keep in the fridge for a few days. Replacing sugary sodas in your day with unsweetened iced black tea is an easy way to eliminate junk calories.

BOBOLI 100% WHOLE WHEAT THIN CRUST PIZZA ROUND

Make your own pizza and make it healthier. This dough delivers 5 grams of fiber per serving, 20 percent of your daily recommendation. Top it with part-skim mozzarella cheese and tomato pasta sauce that's low in sugar.

BROWN RICE

Here's why you should choose brown rice over white rice every chance you get: The milling and polishing process that converts brown rice into white rice destroys 80 percent of the thiamin, 80 percent of the niacin, half of the B_6, 75 percent of the magnesium, 60 percent of the iron, and nearly all of the dietary fiber. For brown rice, only the outermost layer of the hull of the kernel is removed, so it suffers the least damage to its nutritional value. You know that whole grains like brown rice are satiating, but the high-fiber content of brown rice also favorably affects blood glucose levels, which is important for weight loss. Consider this: When Harvard University researchers analyzed the diets of more than 27,000 men over the course of 8 years, they discovered that the men who added one daily serving of whole-grain foods generally weighed 2.5 pounds less than the men who ate only refined-grain foods. One of our favorite instant brown rice products is Uncle Ben's Fast & Natural Whole-Grain Instant Brown Rice. Use it as a side dish or add it to ground meat or poultry for extra body while cutting down on fat.

CRUCIFEROUS VEGETABLES

Broccoli, Brussels sprouts, cauliflower, cabbage, and kale contain cancer-fighting phytochemicals, vitamin C, fiber, and folate. Consumption of these foods seems to be associated with reduced rates of cancers of the lung, colon, and bladder.

DARK CHOCOLATE

It's loaded with antioxidants, many more than its milk chocolate cousin. Plus, milk blocks the absorption of chocolate's antioxidants, so milk chocolate isn't worth the calories. Look for chocolate with 60 percent or higher cocoa content. The darker the chocolate the more antioxidant flavonols and less sugar it has. Watch out, though: Some manufacturers increase the percentage of cocoa by adding extra cocoa butter. When selecting your candy, compare saturated fat counts.

EDAMAME (WHOLE SOY BEANS)

A terrific way to boost fiber and protein while reducing saturated fat is to eat edamame. Soy protein may also help prevent belly fat. Note to self: Snack on salted edamame instead of chips. In addition, a study reported in the *Journal of the American Medical Association* showed that a diet of soy protein, fiber from oats and barley, almonds, and margarine from plant sterols lowered cholesterol as much as statins, the most widely prescribed cholesterol medicine.

EGGS

Calorie for calorie, eggs deliver more biologically usable protein than any other food, including beef. And don't worry about eating the yolk. In addition to protein, it contains vitamin B_{12}, which is necessary for fat breakdown and muscle contraction. Eggs are packed with riboflavin, folate, vitamins B_6, B_{12}, D, and E, and iron, phosphorus, selenium, and zinc. And, no, eating a few a day won't increase your risk of heart disease. If you can find them, buy Eggland's Best eggs. Each egg contains 100 milligrams of heart-healthy omega-3 fats.

EZEKIEL 4:9 SPROUTED WHOLE GRAIN BREAD

This is the best bread you can break. Look up the recipe in the Good Book, Ezekiel 4:9: "Take . . . wheat and barley and beans and lentils and millet and spelt and put them in one vessel and make bread of it." In a sprouted-grain bread, the entire grain sprout is ground into the dough. Here all six of those grains and legumes are sprouted. What you get is nearly the protein equivalent of eggs, containing all nine essential amino acids. Each slice of the bread is just 80 calories and delivers 3 grams of fiber. *Amen.*

FAT FACT
Eating trans fat could double your risk of colon cancer, according to researchers at the University of North Carolina.

FAT-FREE OR LOW-FAT MILK

The beautiful thing about milk is that it has substance, so it helps you feel satisfied quickly and forestalls bingeing. Just keep the Chips Ahoy! away or you'll have a nutritional mutiny on your hands. Here's another terrific thing about milk. A University of Tennessee study found that dieters who consumed between 1,200 and 1,300 milligrams of calcium-rich foods a day lost nearly twice as much weight as those taking in less calcium. Another study in the *Journal of the American College of Nutrition,* which surveyed 1,300 people ages 19 to 38, concluded that increasing intake of calcium and low-fat dairy products may be associated with lower amounts of abdominal fat, particularly in young men.

STEALTH NUTRITION
15 Ways to Sneak More Fiber into Your Diet

The USDA recommends you get 20 to 35 grams of fiber every day. Have you any clue as to how much you are currently eating? You probably have a few more important things on your to-do list. Rest assured that it's pretty tough to get that much fiber while eating the way we typically eat. But you can come really close to, if not hit, those numbers without thinking much and certainly without counting. Just make a handful of these tricks an everyday habit.

● Drop in a handful of berries to add flavor to plain or vanilla yogurt. Half a cup provides 4 grams of fiber.
● Eat the skin of your next baked potato for an extra 2 grams of fiber.
● Pile on the vegetables by layering your sandwich with fresh spinach, tomatoes, sprouts, cucumbers, or peppers.
● Add roughage to chips and salsa by dumping some black or kidney beans into your jarred salsa.
● Choose 100 percent whole-grain bread for your sandwich, and you'll add 3 to 5 grams of fiber per serving.

● Toss ground flaxseeds onto salads or soups for extra bulk and heart-friendly omega-3 fatty acids.
● Blend ½ cup of fresh or frozen fruit into a smoothie. Leave the skins on for up to 4 grams of fiber.
● Watch TV while snacking on 2 cups of low-fat popcorn for 2 grams of fiber.
● Sprinkle garbanzo or kidney beans on your salad. Half a cup delivers up to 6 grams of extra fiber.
● Chomp on raw carrots, broccoli, or pepper strips.
● Stir a fiber supplement containing psyllium into water or juice twice a day, and you'll get an easy 5 grams.
● Crunch on 1 ounce (about a handful) of almonds, peanuts, cashews, pecans, or sunflower seeds for 2 to 4 grams of fiber.
● Top salads or cooked vegetables with ¼ cup of crushed bran cereal or unprocessed wheat bran for an additional 3.5 grams of fiber.
● For dessert, eat dried figs, apricots, or peaches. Add nuts for a fiber-packed trail mix.
● Bite an apple, spread on some almond butter or crunchy natural peanut butter where you just bit. Bite, spread. Repeat.

FLAXSEEDS

One of the few plant sources of healthful omega-3
fatty acids. Toss them into cereal, yogurt, soups, and
stews, and sprinkle them on top of ice cream.

FRUIT

Apples: One apple contains hundreds of phytochemicals, cholesterol-lowering and cancer-fighting nutrients.
Eat the skin. Depending on the variety, apple peels
have up to six times more antioxidants than the flesh
alone. There's truth to the saying that one a day will
keep the doctor away. Researchers from Finland found
that people who eat apples regularly are 27 percent less
likely to develop prediabetes and 25 percent less likely
to have a stroke. Eating one apple before a meal can
help you lose weight, too. Pennsylvania State University researchers found that people who ate an apple
about 15 minutes before lunch consumed almost 190
fewer calories than when they didn't eat an apple. Hey,
but a caramel coating nixes the weight-loss benefits.

Bananas: The combination of a good amount of
potassium and low sodium may help protect against
high blood pressure. Also a top source of vitamin B_6,
bananas may help reduce fatigue, depression, and the
pain of a hangover. Bananas have a creamy texture
often associated with fatty foods, yet they are virtually fat free.

Cherries: Bing cherries have more antioxidants per
serving (a serving is 1 cup) than a cup of red grapes,
half a cup of edamame, or a cup of sliced carrots. The
anti-inflammatory compounds in cherries may help
lower the risk of heart disease as well as arthritis
and cancer.

Grapefruit: The red or pink varieties are slightly
higher in vitamin C than the white. They also contain lycopene, which may reduce the risk of prostate
cancer. But all varieties have natural compounds
called limonoids, which can lower cholesterol.

Kiwifruit: A good source of vitamin C and fiber.

Oranges: All citrus fruits contain anti-inflammatory compounds called flavonoids that may help
prevent cancer. One study even found that these

SUPERSHOT
Mineral Rights

Have a chromium appetizer before you go out for Italian food. In a recent study, Swiss scientists gave men a single 400-microgram (mcg) dose of chromium picolinate before a high-carbohydrate meal. Subsequently, the men's blood glucose levels were 23 percent lower than when they ate the same meal without the supplement. You can find chromium picolinate tablets at GNC and health food stores.

substances work to repair the damaged DNA that leads to cancer growth.

Papayas: If you have a cold, eat a papaya. One medium papaya delivers more than 300 percent of the RDA of vitamin C. The beta-carotene and vitamins C and E in papayas reduce inflammation throughout the body.

Peaches: A solid source of vitamin C for healthy skin and for fighting infection, peaches also have a good amount of dietary fiber to help promote digestive health.

Pears: This fruit is a top source of fiber, vitamin C, and folate, which together can help lower cholesterol, build immunity to infection, and possibly prevent some cancers.

Red grapes: Besides providing protection from heart attack and stroke, antioxidants in red grapes may also help keep your skin flexible and elastic. The resveratrol in red grape skins may help prevent colon cancer, according to researchers at the University of California.

Watermelon: One large wedge provides 9 ounces of water. It's also an excellent source of cancer-fighting lycopene.

GARLIC, ONIONS, CHIVES, SHALLOTS

These breath busters are all cousins, belonging to the alliaceous family. The sulfur compounds found in them fight colon, breast, and lung cancers, and epidemiological studies show that people who consume the most garlic and onions have a lower risk of stomach, colorectal, and prostate cancers. The active compounds in garlic are released when you crush the clove, and they become more robust when sautéed in a little olive oil.

HONEST TEA ORGANIC HONEY GREEN TEA

It packs one of the biggest nutritional punches of all the bottled green teas. It contains 215 milligrams of catechins, ultrapowerful antioxidants that may help prevent cancer, and 71 milligrams of a particularly potent type called EGCG.

HOT PEPPERS

Poblanos, serranos, habaneros, and jalapenos—all chile peppers contain compounds called capsaicinoids, which give them their spicy heat. They are high in carotene and flavonoids and contain more than twice the amount of vitamin C found in citrus fruits.

HUMMUS

This spread made of mashed chickpeas, tahini, and olive oil is rich in protein and fiber. The tahini, a paste made of ground sesame seeds, delivers omega-3 fatty acids. You don't need to eat much; it's filling and high in calories. It makes a terrific high-fiber and protein sandwich spread instead of mayonnaise. For a flavor punch, try Athenos Roasted Garlic hummus.

KASHI GOLEAN AND KASHI HONEY SUNSHINE CEREAL

If you eat a lot of breakfast cereal but are a bit bored by the champions of nutrition, All-Bran and Fiber One, give these cereals a go for a change. GoLean, made with seven whole grains, packs—*get this*—13 grams of protein and 10 grams of dietary fiber. British researchers recently found that people who eat a carbohydrate-rich, high-fiber breakfast before working out burn twice as much fat as they do after a similar meal without all that roughage. If you prefer something a bit sweeter, and especially if you are a Cap'n Crunch fan, try Kashi's Honey Sunshine (6 grams of fiber). The whole-grain yellow corn nuggets resemble Cap'n Crunch cereal and almost taste like it (if you use your imagination), but without all that sugar.

MARANATHA ORGANIC CREAMY & RAW ALMOND BUTTER

Check the ingredients list. It won't take long. "Raw Almonds." That's it. Almond butter is a terrific spread for toast and celery sticks. A 2-tablespoon serving delivers 4 grams of satiating dietary fiber and 7 grams of protein. Of its 16 grams of total fat, just 1 gram is

SUPERSHOT
Get Pickled

Put extra pickles on your next sandwich. Order a side salad with a vinegar-based dressing. Both tactics can counteract the carbohydrate effect of the bread you are eating. In a study, people who consumed acetic acid, the primary component of vinegar and pickle products, with white bread saw their blood glucose dip 23 percent lower than when they ate white bread only.

saturated, and there is no trans fat. But watch your serving size if you are watching calories. Two tablespoons equals 195 calories. You don't need much almond butter to satisfy your hunger.

OATMEAL

You'd be hard pressed to find a better foundation for breakfast. Oatmeal will fill you up with long-burning clean energy. In fact, Pennsylvania State University researchers found that oatmeal keeps insulin levels stable longer than most other foods, which means you won't find yourself craving bagels or candy bars an hour after you eat. Oatmeal, as you know, is rich in fiber. But there are two types: soluble fiber, which acts as a magnet for fluid and digests slower, and insoluble fiber, like that found in vegetables. Oatmeal has a lot of the soluble kind, which is why it has the reputation for clobbering cholesterol. Soluble fiber is believed to reduce your low-density lipoprotein (LDL), the "bad" cholesterol, by binding with digestive acids made from cholesterol and ushering them out of your body. This reduces the absorption of cholesterol in your intestines.

Ten grams or more of soluble fiber a day can decrease your total and LDL cholesterol. Do everything you can to get more soluble fiber into your mouth. Nutritionists recommend more than 25 grams a day, which isn't easy to achieve. But beginning your day with oatmeal is a jump start. You have a couple of choices when it comes to oatmeal. Steel-cut oats, such as *Men's Health*'s favorite Arrowhead Mills Steel Cut Oats, contain more fiber: 2–3 grams more, for a total of 8 grams. The oats are chopped with steel blades, resulting in a chewier oatmeal that's less processed than rolled oats. They'll keep you fuller longer, but they take longer to prepare. If you are pressed for time, the instant oatmeal (rolled oats) is a lot more convenient. But choose the unsweetened, unflavored variety to avoid a lot of sugar. Instead, sweeten your oatmeal with berries, raisins, milk, or a touch of honey.

OLIVE OIL

Olive oil may have a "wimpy" name, but it's a power-house food that controls cravings, helps burn fat, and can even build muscle. Olive oil is a monounsaturated fat that has been associated with everything from lower rates of heart disease and colon cancer to a reduced risk of diabetes and osteoporosis. You've heard about that for years. But it also appears that olive oil prevents muscle breakdown by lowering levels of a cellular protein that is linked to muscle wasting and weakness. Tip: Choose the extra-virgin olive oil, which has higher levels of the antioxidant vitamin E.

PORK CHOPS

Per gram of protein, pork chops contain almost five times the selenium—an essential mineral that's linked to a lower risk of prostate cancer—of beef, and twice that of chicken. And researchers have found that a 6-ounce serving daily helped people preserve their muscle while losing weight.

PUMPKIN SEEDS

Did you know that men with the highest levels of magnesium in their blood have a 40 percent lower risk of early death than those with the lowest levels? That's why you should eat pumpkin seeds. Roasted pumpkin seeds contain 150 milligrams of magnesium per ounce. Most men don't get enough magnesium in their daily diets. Add pumpkin seeds regularly and you'll likely hit that daily target of 420 milligrams. Eat them whole; the shells provide extra fiber.

QUINOA

This nutty-tasting grain has about twice the protein of regular cereal grains, fewer carbohydrates, and even some healthful fats. It's considered a "complete" protein, like eggs, because it contains all of the essential amino acids your body needs for muscle growth. Quinoa can be used to make pilafs, risottos, salads, and soups. Find it in the rice aisle or the health food section of your grocery store.

SARDINES

This delicious cold-water fish delivers some of the highest amounts of omega-3 fatty acids and protein of any food. Not only is fish oil an anti-inflammatory agent, it also helps protect against heart arrhythmias. And a single can of sardines has more calcium than a cup of whole milk (because you eat the bones). Omega-3s help suppress the activity of prostaglandins and leukotrienes, which can activate various diseases, including blood clots and joint inflammation. They also help protect the immune system.

SMART BALANCE OMEGA PEANUT BUTTER

This spread has no trans fat and each serving supplies 1,000 milligrams of omega-3 fats. That's like eating six sardines.

SUNFLOWER SEEDS

If you want to look younger, eat sunflower seeds. They have the highest natural vitamin E content of any other food around. "No antioxidant is more effective at fighting the aging effects of free radicals," says Barry Swanson, PhD, a professor of food science at Washington State University.

SWEET POTATOES

These are higher in fiber and lower in carbohydrates than white potatoes. Here's another reason to love them. They, too, may help you look younger. European researchers recently found that pigments from beta-carotene-rich foods like sweet potatoes and

---

SUPERSHOT
A Coffee to Go

A shot of espresso or a couple cups of coffee prior to a workout may help you work harder. A study published in *Medicine and Science in Sports and Exercise* found that men who drank 2½ cups of coffee a few hours before an exercise test were able to sprint 9 percent longer than when they didn't drink any. (It's believed the caffeine directly stimulates the muscles.) Caveat: Please skip this Supershot if you have high blood pressure.

carrots can build up in your skin, helping to prevent ultraviolet rays from prematurely aging skin.

THOMAS' HEARTY GRAINS 100% WHOLE WHEAT BAGEL

Great tasting and made with 100 percent whole wheat, it won't spike your blood sugar the way a regular bagel can.

TOMATOES

According to the FDA, eating tomatoes may reduce the risk of prostate, gastric, and pancreatic cancers, thanks to their high concentration of the nutrient lycopene. You don't have to eat fresh tomatoes to reap the benefits: Pasta and pizza sauces deliver it, too, since cooking doesn't reduce lycopene's potency.

NUTS

In a study of more than 3,000 African American men and women, those who ate nuts at least five times a week cut their risk of dying of heart disease by 44 percent compared with people who ate nuts less frequently. Most nuts are the perfect snack food, packed with muscle-building protein, filling fiber, and heart-healthy monounsaturated fats. Numerous studies have shown that almonds, Brazil nuts, hazelnuts, macadamia nuts, peanuts, pistachios, pecans, and walnuts all reduce levels of LDL cholesterol. Walnuts, in particular, have a keen effect on lowering not only LDL cholesterol but also lipoprotein(a), a compound that increases clotting and can lead to a stroke, according to a study published in *Annals of Internal Medicine*. Pistachios have a relaxing effect on arteries and blood pressure. Pennsylvania State University nutritionists found that subjects who ate a handful daily for 1 month kept their blood pressure down in stressful situations.

SUPERSHOT
The Whey
to Eat Less

Drinking a shake made from whey protein about 2 hours before dinner can prevent you from overeating. When University of Toronto scientists presented 22 men with an all-you-can-eat pizza buffet, the men who had consumed a whey protein drink 2 hours earlier ate about 200 calories fewer than men who drank a soy- or egg-based protein shake. The researchers say it's because whey triggers the release of several gut peptides that promote satiety.

WILD SALMON

This fish is rich in the omega-3 fatty acid DHA. People with the highest blood levels of this nutrient have a 47 percent lower chance of developing dementia, according to a study published in the *Archives of Neurology*. DHA, a component of neurons, plays a key role in memory and learning. It's best to eat wild salmon rather than farmed fish; the farmed salmon may not get the appropriate marine diet needed to produce high amounts of omega-3s.

YOGURT

Yogurt is one of the few foods that contain conjugated linoleic acid, a special type of fat that some studies show can reduce body fat. And if you're exercising hard, this stuff delivers a perfect combination of protein and carbohydrates for workout recovery and muscle growth.

REAL GUYS—REAL RESULTS

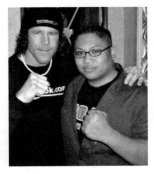

BEFORE:
280
POUNDS

AFTER:
153
POUNDS

"My life was spinning out of control."

VITALS: Medwin Mina, 31, San Francisco, CA
OCCUPATION: Sales manager
HEIGHT: 5'8"
LESSON LEARNED: Little changes, like parking a bit farther way, let you ease into exercise.

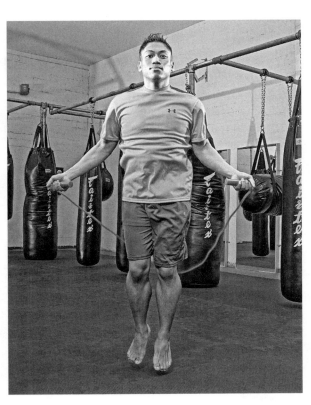

Mina kept active in high school as a tennis player, and his parents provided him with healthy, home-cooked meals. But that reliance on Dad's cooking left him at a loss when he went to college. "I began living off fast food," says Mina. With the value menu as his guide, he reached 280 pounds by his junior year.

THE TURNING POINT

Mina's low point came during a trip to an amusement park with friends. "I tried to sit in the seat of a roller coaster and couldn't get my harness to fit," he says. The next day, he tossed out his fried foods and replaced them with healthier options, such as fruits, vegetables, and baked chicken. Then he enrolled in a 5-day-a-week martial-arts class. After a year of punching, kicking, and face-to-face battles, Mina had shed 100 pounds.

LIFE IN THE FIT LANE

Mina starts his day with a 3- to 5-mile run. At night, he works out for 2 hours by jumping rope, shadowboxing, and sparring. To fuel his new lifestyle, Mina relies on high-protein meals but allows himself a few old favorites on occasion. "I've learned that I can eat what I want, as long as I keep it in moderation," he says.

THE REWARD

Mina now loves to hit the open water in a kayak and enjoys other outdoor activities like hiking. "I've grown to love exercising outdoors, since I'm not worried about becoming winded anymore," he says. Even better, his new lifestyle helped him drop a 10-year smoking habit.

MINA'S BEST BELLY OFF! TIPS

• Find a sport you love. If the activity doesn't feel like work, exercise comes naturally.
• Set a bigger goal. Mini-goals are important, but setting a larger overall goal can keep you on message.
• Eat what you enjoy. Don't deprive yourself. Keep your favorite foods, but gradually reduce the portions so you cut back on fat and calories.

41 SMART BELLY OFF! FOOD SWAPS
Trim Calories by Making the Right Choices

Cutting out 500 calories a day adds up to a pound of weight loss in a week. That's even before you lace up your running shoes. And it's easy to do. Just make a few simple swaps in your diet and you'll hit 500 or more without feeling that you sacrificed at all. Try these this week.

CHOOSE	INSTEAD OF	CALORIES SAVED
Carbohydrates		
Whole-grain English muffin with 1 tablespoon blueberry fruit spread	Blueberry muffin	270
$1/2$ whole-wheat bagel	Plain bagel	90
Whole-grain pita	Hamburger bun	55
$1/2$ large baked potato	1 cup mashed potatoes	100
1 slice whole-grain toast topped with $1/2$ banana mashed with 1 teaspoon peanut butter	1-inch-thick slice banana bread	260
$1/2$ cup oatmeal	$1/2$ cup granola	125
$1/2$ cup brown rice mixed with $1/2$ cup frozen vegetables and 1 teaspoon olive oil	$1/2$ cup white rice with 2 teaspoons butter	65
$1/2$ cup whole-wheat spaghetti, $1/4$ cup sliced mushrooms, $1/2$ cup marinara sauce	1 cup spaghetti with $1/2$ cup meat sauce	160
Fats/Condiments		
1 teaspoon olive oil	1 tablespoon butter	60
Cooking spray in a nonstick skillet	Butter or margarine	100
1 tablespoon all-natural peanut butter	2 tablespoons peanut butter	85
Balsamic vinaigrette made with 1 tablespoon flaxseed oil and 1 tablespoon balsamic vinegar	$1/4$ cup blue cheese dressing	175
1 teaspoon olive oil mixed with $1/2$ teaspoon mustard and a dash of salt and pepper on sandwiches or tuna	2 tablespoons mayonnaise	165
$1/8$ mashed avocado with lemon juice, salt, pepper	2 tablespoons cream cheese	55
$1/4$ cup hummus	$1/4$ cup ranch dip for vegetables	190
Snacks		
Sliced raw vegetables	Tortilla chips with salsa	100
Pizza topped with sliced grilled chicken	Pizza topped with pepperoni	100
4 (1-inch) squares of dark chocolate	1 large chocolate chip cookie	180
$1/2$ cup ice cream with 1 cup sliced strawberries	1 cup ice cream alone	100

CHOOSE	INSTEAD OF	CALORIES SAVED
Snacks (cont.)		
$^1/_2$ cup unshelled pistachios	$^1/_2$ cup Peanut M&Ms	90
Baked tortilla chips, 1-oz bag	Tortilla chips, 1-oz bag	50
2 cups air-popped popcorn	1 cup potato chips (about 15)	95
$^1/_2$ cup diced strawberries with $^1/_2$ cup fat-free vanilla yogurt	1 cup fruit-on-bottom yogurt	105
Drinks		
Water with a squeeze of lemon	16 oz soda	180
12 oz light beer	16 oz beer	100
12 oz latte made with fat-free milk	16 oz latte made with whole milk	120
16 oz iced coffee made with fat-free milk	16 oz iced Mocha Frappuccino	270
$^1/_2$ cup juice cut with $^1/_2$ cup water	1 cup juice	60
Dairy		
1 tablespoon Parmesan cheese	$^1/_4$ cup grated Cheddar cheese	90
$^1/_2$ cup reduced-fat mozzarella	$^1/_2$ cup grated whole mozzarella	85
8 oz fat-free milk	8 oz 2% milk	50
$^1/_2$ cup part-skim ricotta cheese	$^1/_2$ cup whole-milk ricotta cheese	45
3 large egg whites	2 large eggs	95
Protein		
3 oz skinless chicken breast	3 oz chicken breast with skin	30
3 oz filet mignon	3 oz New York strip	60
3 oz tuna steak	3 oz rib eye	55
3 oz turkey meatloaf	3 oz beef meat loaf	115
Lean ground turkey burger	Ground beef burger	85
2 slices turkey bacon	2 slices pork bacon	25
3 oz pork tenderloin	4 oz pork chop	100
$^1/_2$ cup pinto beans	1 cup refried beans	135

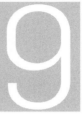

50 WAYS TO LEAVE YOUR BLUBBER

How to Boil, Sauté, Roast, and Chop Your Way to Fewer Calories, Less Fat and More Nutrients

W**HEN I FACE ANY DIFFICULT CHALLENGE,** like trying to get my kids to eat their lima beans, I take comfort in Pete Seeger's folk tune *Step by Step*. Know it? Let me sing it for you:

Step by step the longest march can be won, can be won.
Many stones can form an arch, singly none, singly none.
And by union what we will can be accomplished still.
Drops of water turn a mill, singly none, singly none.

That chorus about the value of diligence and taking small steps holds the secret to making anything worthwhile happen, from learning to play the guitar to bouncing

FIT FACT
Knowing that some foods are unhealthy takes away from the pleasure of eating them, say University of Mississippi researchers studying people who checked restaurant nutrition guides before ordering.

back from a job loss. It certainly applies to the challenges of losing weight and getting back in shape. Sure, it's not a revolutionary notion by any means. Heck, Seeger borrowed those words from a poem that graced the cover of the 1864 constitution of the American Miners' Association. But it's smart. And it works.

Have you hit a plateau? Are the pounds slower to come off these days? Are your muscles sore? Do you feel like blowing off your workout and diving into stuffed-crust pizza with pepperoni? All that's normal. You might download a copy of Seeger's *Step by Step* and put it in heavy rotation on your iPod. Then try these 50 smart ways to turbocharge your weight-loss efforts. When it comes to cooking and eating, tiny tweaks can add up to more pounds lost and another notch on your belt.

1. SLICE YOUR STEAK, EAT LESS

Slicing thinly will make your portions seem bigger and more satisfying. In a recent study at Japan's National Food Research Institute, participants who compared equal amounts of sliced and whole vegetables rated the sliced piles up to 27 percent larger. When you *believe* you're eating a larger portion of food, you may trick yourself into feeling more satisfied with fewer calories.

2. KNOW YOUR DELI MEATS

Sandwiches are the architecture of the common man, but you need to start with a solid foundation. The hierarchy of health, in descending order:

- Turkey and chicken
- Roast beef
- Ham
- Weird processed things like salami and olive loaf

For example, instead of an Italian submarine sandwich with cheese and mixed cold cuts like salami and bologna, choose a roast beef hero, and you can trim your fat intake by up to 30 percent.

3. DON'T RUIN A TUNA

Mayonnaise will turn your tuna sandwich into a fatty disaster. Instead of mixing in a lot of mayo, squeeze lemon juice and add pepper and hot sauce to your tuna. It tastes great.

4. GET *GRATER* TASTE FROM LESS CHEESE

Get yourself a good grater. Use it to grate a piece of Parmesan or other hard cheese on your sandwich, and you'll save a lot of fat calories compared to standard sliced fare as long as you add a sprinkling for flavor rather than an avalanche of grated cheese.

5. EMBARGO THE OIL

When grilling chicken, try this oil-free marinade: Combine 3 cups of apple juice and two cloves of pressed garlic with 1 cup of reduced-sodium soy sauce.

6. MAKE LEANER BUFFALO WINGS

Make some spicy low-fat buffalo wings. Instead of using chicken wings, make them with skinless chicken-breast tenders. Marinate them overnight in a mixture of Louisiana hot sauce, olive oil, lots of garlic powder, and red wine vinegar. (Experiment with the amounts to suit your taste.) Then roast the chicken "wings" at 400°F for 15 minutes.

7. TOP A TATER

If you love baked potatoes, you don't have to give them up just because of their high glycemic load rating. Keep your blood sugar levels balanced by adding a topping, like Cheddar cheese, mushrooms, broccoli, and spinach.

8. STUFF YOUR BURGERS

Scoop a hole in the middle of your burger before grilling, and fill it with olives, mushrooms, or any vegetable you like. This makes the recommended serving of beef (3 ounces) look and feel like a massive hunk of burger, when it's much leaner than that.

9. RINSE YOUR BEANS

Canned beans—kidney, cannellini, chickpeas—are a quick and easy way to add protein and fiber to your meals. But they can also spike your daily sodium intake, increasing your risk of stomach cancer and high blood pressure. Simply rinsing them, however, will shed one-third of their sodium.

10. SHAKE ON OREGANO

One tablespoon of fresh oregano has the same antioxidant power as an entire apple, according to researchers at the U.S. Department of Agriculture. Mexican oregano has the highest count, but Italian oregano and Greek mountain oregano trail closely behind. One of the most versatile herbs, oregano can be added to anything from noodles to meats to salad dressings.

11. CATCH UP ON YOUR LYCOPENE

Squirt some organic ketchup on that bun. Researchers at the Agricultural Research Service in California found that organic ketchups have about twice as much cancer-fighting lycopene as the regular varieties. A simple visual clue you've got the correct ketchup? Organic varieties are a slightly darker shade of red than regular ketchups.

FAT FACT
Eating more than four slices of white bread a day may double your risk of developing kidney cancer, according to a study of the diet records of 2,300 people.

12. GIVE IN TO CHOCOLATE CRAVINGS

You don't have to deprive yourself of the sweet stuff. Shave dark chocolate into savory dishes like chili and barbecue sauces—you'll add a rich flavor along with flavonoids. They can lower your risk of heart disease and keep your cholesterol in check. And shaving ensures you don't go overboard on the dark. Or try this for a nighttime snack: Melt 2 tablespoons of chocolate chips in the microwave and swirl that into 4 ounces of vanilla yogurt. Top with a tablespoon of slivered almonds.

13. MAKE IT MEATLESS

Next time you're hankering for a veal Parmesan sandwich, try this vegetarian hot Italian sub. Brown some cubed eggplant pieces under a broiler with a little olive oil. Then mix with tomato sauce and capers. Place in a kaiser roll. Top with grated Parmesan. Fat savings: 18 grams.

14. CURRY FAVOR WITH YOGURT

Replace the high-fat coconut milk in your curries with low-fat plain yogurt. The yogurt adds that creamy texture without the extra fat from the coconut.

15. DO YOUR OWN DIPS

Make dips healthier by using fat-free sour cream or yogurt. Mix in an equal part of salsa, the hotter the better. Jazz it up with lemon, dried herbs, whatever.

16. SQUASH THE FAT

Replace half of the Cheddar in quesadillas, mac 'n' cheese, or grilled cheese sandwiches with pureed butternut squash. This significantly lowers the fat and calorie counts, won't compromise the taste, and gives you a slew of added vitamins and heart-healthy potassium.

17. PACK A PITA

Add extra vegetables to your next sandwich by packing them in a whole-wheat pita pocket rather than between conventional slices of bread. Pitas simply hold more.

18. STIR-FRY RIGHT

Let your vegetables stir-fry in their own moisture instead of an oil bath. Add a few drops of oil to start, and then use water rather than more oil as you're stir-frying.

19. ADD CHEESE TO BREAKFAST

Grate hard, flavorful cheese, like Parmesan, on hot cereals and oatmeal for added protein and flavor. "The key is to add protein to *all* meals, as it fills you up faster and may help you burn more calories," says Milton Stokes, RD, of the American Dietetic Association.

20. WARM UP YOUR OIL

Heat your skillet before adding oil, and less fat will be absorbed by the food. Warm oil cooks more efficiently; cold oil tends to soak into meats and vegetables.

21. WRAP MEATS IN GREENS

To cut carbs, ditch the sandwich bread and do as the Koreans do: Wrap spicy cooked beef or chicken with leafy greens. Try Chinese cabbage, bok choy, or romaine lettuce. Replacing two slices of bread with one large lettuce leaf saves you about 30 grams of carbohydrate.

22. START A MEAL WITH A WATER APPETIZER

Drink two glasses of water before every meal. This will keep you hydrated and make you feel less hungry, possibly reducing your food intake and aiding weight loss.

23. GIVE YOUR PANCAKES A NUTRITIONAL BOOST

Next time you make pancakes, replace ¼ cup of flour with ¼ cup of cornmeal. It'll give your pancakes great texture, and the cornmeal will add extra fiber and magnesium to an otherwise rather nutritionally vacant breakfast.

24. ALWAYS SAY "ICED TEA"

Get into the healthy habit. When the waitress asks what you want to drink, always say "iced tea—unsweetened." You'll cut calories and earn a dose of antioxidants, which are crucial to your body's defense against heart disease, cancer, even wrinkles. A U.S. Department of Agriculture study found that a serving of black tea had more flavonoids than a serving of broccoli or carrots.

25. GO HALFSIES

Here's a simple rule for buffet eating at a party that'll help you keep your meal balanced for weight loss: Fill half of your plate with vegetables and fruit. Fill the rest of your plate with equal amounts of whole grains and other high-fiber carbs, and lean protein.

26. CREATE THE BEST STEAM ROOM FOR YOUR BROCCOLI

For perfectly cooked *and* nutrient-rich vegetables, rinse, throw them in a sealed container, and micro-wave for 3 or 4 minutes. Boiling, blanching, or over-steaming zaps vegetables of their nutrients—the only water you need are the drops that cling after rinsing.

27. BUILD A BETTER PIZZA

Can't resist pepperoni? Go for it, but help offset the damage by ordering two or more vegetable top-pings for every meat topping. Since the carcinogens in processed meats such as pepperoni and sausage increase your cancer risk with every serving, accord-ing to the American Institute for Cancer Research, load on a variety of vegetables—green peppers, onions—that can help protect against cancer.

IT WORKS FOR ME

"I pack my next day's lunch right after I eat dinner. Because I'm not hungry anymore, it tricks me into not bringing as much food for lunch."

—Michael Young, Laguna Niguel, CA, who lost 33 pounds

28. REPRISE *BLAZING SADDLES*

If all you have is instant white rice, just add a can of beans. The beans lessen the effect that the starchy white rice will have on your blood sugar.

29. BE SLICK WITH YOUR OIL

"Avoid splashing 'light' olive oils over your salads," says Elena Paravantes, registered dietitian for the Hellenic Dietetic Association in Greece—they have fewer cancer-fighting antioxidants than the extra-virgin kind, plus they have a less intense flavor. Not sure if your oil's up to snuff? "Good quality extra-virgin olive oil should have a fruity, peppery, slightly bitter taste and leave a faint burning sensation on the throat," she says.

SUPERSHOT
The Ultimate Muscle Shake

A cocktail of protein, carbs, and creatine can help you build muscle faster, according to Australian researchers. Men who consumed a mix of 40 grams each of carbs and protein, plus 5 grams of creatine, during 10 weeks of weight training packed on 68 percent more muscle than those who took in only protein and carbs. Study author Alan Hayes, PhD, attributes the muscle growth to the creatine, which he says helps lifters train harder and recover faster.

30. BULK UP YOUR MEATBALLS

Grate carrots, squash, or zucchini into any meatball mixture. They add bulk, moisture, and vitamins but don't alter that meaty flavor you're after.

31. TURN YOUR SANDWICHES GREEN

Replace mayo with a spread of ripe avocado to moisten a dry sandwich. Avocados are packed with monounsaturated (good) fat to help lower your cholesterol. Plus, researchers at Ohio State University found that phytochemicals in avocados may help prevent mouth cancer.

32. CHOOSE THE BLUES

Use blue corn tortillas in your next batch of nachos, fajitas, or quesadillas for more effective weight loss. A team of Mexican and Venezuelan researchers found that tortillas made from blue corn have a lower glycemic load than white corn tortillas do, so they won't raise your blood sugar as quickly. The blue variety also has more protein and less starch.

33. BRING THE HEAT

Scientists at the University of Tasmania in Australia found that overweight people are more likely to slim down after consuming a meal that contains chile peppers than one that isn't on fire. Capsaicin, the chemical that makes chiles hot, may help the liver clear insulin—the hormone that tells your body to store fat—from the bloodstream after a meal.

34. TRY THIS SPIN ON A GYRO

For a low-fat gyro, mix some fat-free yogurt with chopped or sliced cucumbers, add a squeeze of lemon juice, and pour over a pita stuffed with grilled chicken or beef strips.

35. THICKEN YOUR SIDE DISHES

Replace the whole milk in your mashed potatoes with evaporated fat-free milk. It's lower in fat and higher in calcium per cup, and still manages to add richness to your mash. You'll find it in a can—usually near baking products.

36. SWAP RED MEAT FOR RED LENTILS

To make a low-fat, antioxidant-packed lasagna, use half the usual amount of ground meat and make up the difference with red lentils. They're still protein packed, but lentils are fat-free and high in fiber, making them more filling, too. And since red lentils have a neutral taste, they'll simply soak up the flavors in your sauce. You won't even notice them. Promise.

37. REVISE YOUR REUBEN

Simulate a cheese Reuben by replacing fatty corned beef with turkey ham and topping it with low-fat mozzarella, mustard, spicy shredded cabbage, and pickles. Slap all that on traditional rye bread and broil until the cheese melts. Fat savings: 10 grams.

IT WORKS FOR ME

"Portion control is my secret weapon. I eat a lot of things I love, but in moderation."

—Matt Carnignan, Bow, NH, who lost 90 pounds

38. TRADE CRACKERS FOR OATS

For any meat recipe that calls for crackers or bread crumbs, use an equal amount of rolled oats instead. This ramps up your soluble fiber intake, which can help lower your cholesterol. Use the quick-cooking variety of oatmeal because it retains moisture well and doesn't alter the meaty taste.

39. KEEP YOUR ABS HARD WITH SOFT CHEESE

Use softer cheeses like goat, feta, and ricotta on pizzas and sandwiches because they're naturally about a third lower in fat and calories than harder cheeses. And when you need the full-fat cheeses, go for strong flavors like Parmesan, blue, and extra-sharp Cheddar—you'll get the same great taste but with less cheese.

40. GO FRY A COD

To soften some of the damage inflicted by Britain's national treasure, try this healthier DIY version of fish-and-chips—courtesy of Mark and Pete Petrou of Petrou Brothers in Cambridgeshire, England, 2006's National Fish-and-Chip Shop of the Year:

1. Buy fillets or loins of white fish such as haddock or cod, and cut into strips.
2. Make a light tempura-like batter by mixing iced sparkling water with self-rising flour.
3. Dust the fish strips with self-rising flour and roll in the tempura batter.
4. Shallow fry the strips in hot canola oil, which is loaded with good fats: Fill one-third of your pan with oil and heat it to about 350°F. Fry the fish until crispy. (Use a thermometer!)
5. For the chips: Cut potatoes into your preferred size and toss them in 1 to 2 tablespoons of canola oil with salt, herbs, garlic—anything you want, really. Then bake them at 450°F for about 30 minutes.

41. PREVENT BLOOD SUGAR SPIKES WITH VINEGAR

Start a meal with a salad or vegetables drizzled with a vinaigrette dressing. Arizona State University nutritionists believe that the acetic acid in vinegar interferes with enzymes that break down carbohydrates. A few teaspoons of vinegar per meal can keep blood sugar levels from rising quickly.

42. FREEZE YOUR BANANAS

That way they will always be on hand for use in a smoothie. And because they are naturally sweet, you won't need any sugar.

43. EAT THE CRUMBS

If you're baking something with a topping of grated cheese, cut fat by halving the cheese and replacing with whole-wheat bread crumbs. This mimics the crispy texture of baked cheese and adds fiber.

44. SLIM YOUR CHICKEN SALAD

Use thick, Greek-style plain yogurt to cut down on the amount of mayo you need to make chicken, tuna, or egg salad sandwiches.

45. KEEP A LITTLE SHRIMP ON HAND

For an easy way to add lean protein to your meals, stock up on frozen shrimp. It defrosts in just 15 minutes under cold running water. And with the cooked variety, you have an instant healthy snack. If uncooked, throw it into your pasta sauces, stir-fries, or noodle soups in the last 5 minutes.

46. SHELL YOUR NUTS

Buy nuts in their shells. More time shelling equals less time shoveling handfuls into your mouth.

SUPERSHOT
Oil Your Appetite

Fifteen minutes before dinner, soak up 2 teaspoons of olive oil with half a slice of wheat bread or the end of a crusty baguette and eat it to control your appetite. The olive oil will stimulate the release of a hormone in your stomach called cholecystokinin, which signals the brain to stop eating. It'll help you eat less during dinner or skip dessert.

47. . . . BUT, BOIL THEM FIRST

Boil your peanuts (in their shells) for about 3 hours. Researchers at Alabama A&M University found that boiled peanuts—a popular snack food in China, Southeast Asia, Australia, and the southern United States—have up to four times more antioxidants than raw, dry, or roasted peanuts.

48. POUR A SECOND ROUND

The typical bottled soft drink contains 2 to 2.5 servings, but of course, it's common to drink the whole bottle in a sitting. Cut your calories in half by pouring half the bottle into a glass to drink now and putting the rest of the bottle in the fridge.

49. DOUBLE THE ORDER

Always order your pizza with double tomato sauce and low-fat cheese. Reducing the mozzarella by just one third will save you 20 grams of fat. That's as much as in a McDonald's Quarter Pounder. And if you double the sauce on your pizza, you get double the lycopene. Having a sandwich? Order double tomato slices. Another chance for a healthy dose of lycopene.

50. LEAVE NO CHEERIO BEHIND

To get all of the vitamins out of your cereal, drink the milk left in the bowl. You've admirably resisted the Frosted Flakes in favor of a less sugary breakfast cereal that's fortified with vitamins, but that doesn't mean you're actually getting all of the nutrients listed on the side of the box. Up to 40 percent of the vitamins in your cereal dissolve into that orphaned puddle of milk. Drink up.

REAL GUYS—REAL RESULTS

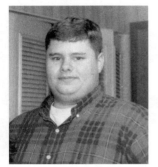

BEFORE:
317
POUNDS

AFTER:
173
POUNDS

"I feel as if I can accomplish anything now."

VITALS: Andrew Staton, 34, Rehoboth Beach, DE
OCCUPATION: Real estate agent
HEIGHT: 5'9"
LESSON LEARNED: Diet isn't a short-term regimen; it's a lifestyle.

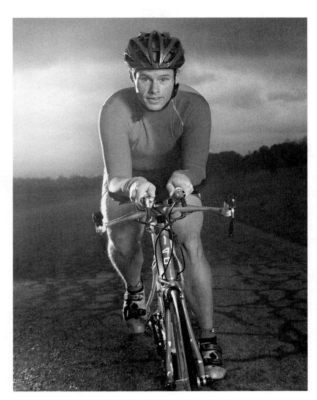

Staton never knew what it was like to be athletic. "I was a fat kid, a fat teenager, and a fat adult," he says. He passed the 300-pound mark after college, as his career took off and his activity level plummeted. That's when Staton realized his weight was holding him down professionally, too.

THE TURNING POINT

Staton remembers the day he took control of his weight. "I just woke up and thought, I'm going to get a hold of my life," he says. Staton halved his calorie intake, hit the elliptical trainer for an hour a day, 6 days a week, and watched the first 60 pounds melt away. He soon moved his workouts from the gym to the road, and just 7 months later, ran his first 10-K. Two years later, he completed the Marine Corps Marathon. "When people notice your weight loss, it gives you a high that drives you forward," he says.

LIFE IN THE FIT LANE

Staton's road to weight loss didn't end with the marathon. "You have to do absolutely everything you did to lose the weight to keep it off," Staton says. That means keeping portions small—a slice of whole-wheat toast with peanut butter for breakfast, a low-calorie lunch, and a dinner of lean meat, a side, and salad. It's all quickly burned off in exercise: Staton typically logs 9 hours of cardio and an hour of weight training a week.

THE REWARD

Staton found that his trim physique conveyed dedication and perseverance, and his real estate business boomed. At the same time, his athletic goals continued to shoot upward. Last summer, Staton competed in his first Ironman triathlon. Next, he plans to repeat the feat in Switzerland. "This one is all about speed," Staton says. "I'm hoping to finish in under 13 hours."

STATON'S BEST BELLY OFF! TIPS
● Use common sense. Fast food and candy will make you fat. It's not rocket science.
● Rotate your training intensity. Give yourself one recovery week a month.
● Set a near-impossible goal. Nothing motivates you like facing a 140.6-mile race.

PART IV

Making the Belly Off! Diet Work for You

10

THE CORE WORKOUT
Improve Your Life While Finding Your Abs

YOU MAY THINK that sporting a six-pack of abdominal muscles is an impossible dream. (We beg to differ.) Or maybe sculpting rippling abs just doesn't make your top ten list of life's priorities. That's cool. You can be fit without looking like Michelangelo's *David*. But that doesn't mean you earn a pass on an abdominal workout. It's a required course on the syllabus of the Belly Off! Diet. Not because abs exercises will melt your gut (they really won't), but because you never know when there will be a sale on 15-ounce cans of stewed tomatoes at ShopRite.

Let me explain. It was an incredible deal: two-for-one on stewed tomatoes with Italian spices during the grocery chain's "can-can" event. We stocked up. Filled a box with those cans.

And when I lifted that box out of the Volvo, my hips turned to walk away while my upper body hung back under the weight of the cans. *Ping!* The muscle pull in my lower back kept me out of the gym for 2 weeks. I was popping 600 milligrams of prescription ibuprofen and hobbling around like a 90-year-old man who had misplaced his walker.

You see my point. If I had been doing my abs exercises, I might have avoided wrenching my back to save $4.35 on stewed tomatoes. Abs exercises are the defense against the flea-flicker plays of modern life. Think about it. Every movement you make originates from your center of gravity, the core muscles of your torso, which include the abdominals, obliques, and the pelvis and back muscles. Lift a kid. Thank your core muscles, not your biceps. Rise out of bed. Thank your core. Do the twist or the horizontal bop. High-five your abs. Core is key whether you're sitting, dancing, or having sex. And if you want more power in your golf swing, baseball pitch, or tennis serve, you have to go to the source: your core.

Before we start conditioning our core, let's review the biomechanics of this pivotal area. Your core is much more than your abs. It's actually composed of four separate muscle groups—the *rectus abdominis,* the *external* and *internal obliques,* and the *transverse abdominis.*

Rectus Abdominis. Running from your breastbone to your pubic bone, this is the muscle responsible for the six-pack look. It is what we typically mean when we talk about the "abs." It helps flex the spinal column and is active during forward movements, like crunches. During side bending motions, these muscles help to stabilize the trunk.

External and Internal Obliques. Located on each side of the rectus abdominis, the fibers of these muscles run diagonally across your midsection. The obliques work together to rotate your torso from side to side, they allow sideways bending, and contribute to compression of the abdomen.

Transverse Abdominis. This deep layer of abdominal muscles wraps around the torso from front to back like a weight belt. It stabilizes the spine, protects the internal organs, and helps with breathing.

Hip Flexors. While they're technically not abdominal muscles, the hip flexors play a crucial rule in many core exercise movements. They are made up of two muscle groups. One attaches your pelvis to your thighbones, and the other attaches your lower back to your thighbones. Together they are responsible for drawing your legs to your midsection.

There are dozens and dozens of moves that exercise your abs, so you should never get bored with these babies. Choose five to do in a circuit. By circuit, we mean performing different exercises one after another with little or no rest between sets. Circuit training is terrific for cardiovascular fitness and for keeping workouts short. When selecting your five exercises, include one move that targets each part of your core.

For starters, try the terrific five-move core circuit starting on page 258. Begin by doing 1 set of 10 to 20 repetitions of each move two to three times a week. After 2 weeks, switch in some of the other abs exercises at the end of this chapter or the dozens you'll find at menshealth.com/bellyoff. Changing the angle of the stress through different exercises keeps your abs challenged, so they'll grow stronger and firmer. When one circuit becomes too easy, gradually increase to three full circuits. Tip: Do your abs circuit at the beginning of your bodyweight or lifting workouts and you'll be less likely to blow them off because you are tired or out of time.

SUPERSHOT
Tough Love

Squeeze a tennis ball as hard as you can while you do crunches. This causes radiational tension, which allows you to contract your abs more forcefully.

CORE CIRCUIT

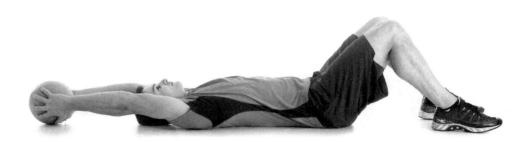

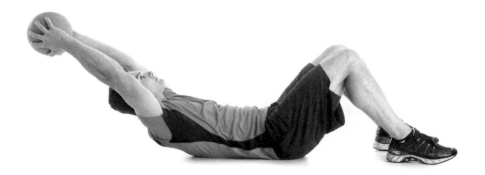

LONG-ARM WEIGHTED CRUNCH (UPPER ABS)

You're already familiar with the traditional crunch. Get into that position with your knees bent and feet flat on the floor. Hold either a light medicine ball in your hands or a light dumbbell in each hand and extend your arms straight back behind your head. Now crunch forward, keeping your arms straight. Do the crunch slowly to avoid generating momentum with your arms, and remember to keep your arms straight overhead throughout the exercise.

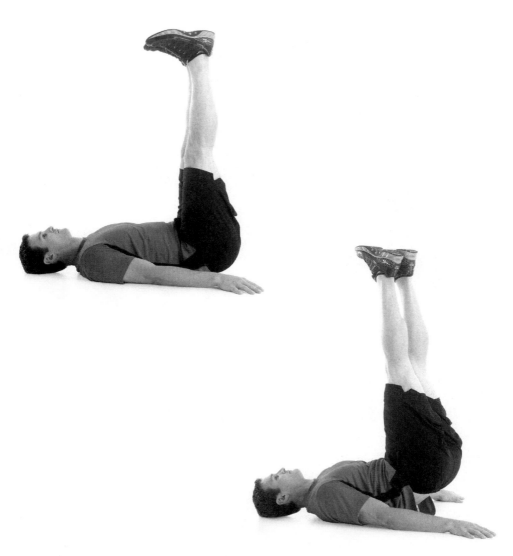

CORKSCREW (LOWER ABS AND OBLIQUES)

Lie on your back with your legs raised directly over your hips. Your
knees should be slightly bent. Place your hands at your sides, palms
down. Use your lower abs to raise your hips off the floor and toward
your rib cage, elevating your feet straight up. Simultaneously twist
your hips to the right. Hold for a second, and then return to the
starting position. Repeat the exercise, this time twisting to the left.

CORE CIRCUIT

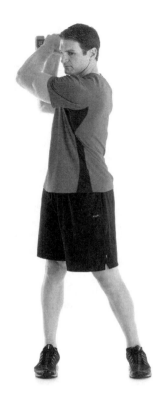

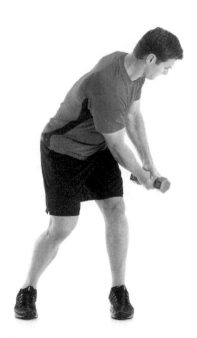

WOOD CHOP (OBLIQUES)

Stand with your feet shoulder-width apart and your hands holding a light dumbbell next to your right ear. Now rotate your torso to the left as you extend your arms and lower the dumbbell to the outside of your left knee. Wood chop, get it? Repeat for 10–20 reps. Switch sides, starting with the dumbbell at your left ear and move it toward the outside of your right knee. Chop slowly and under control, to avoid allowing the momentum of the dumbbell to wrench your back.

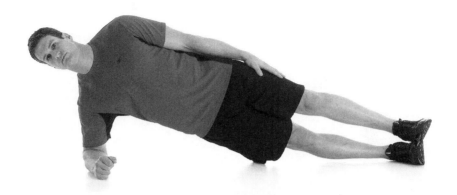

SIDE BRIDGE (TRANSVERSE ABDOMINIS)

Lie on your right side with your forearm on the floor under your shoulder to prop you up. Stack your feet. Now, contract your core muscles and press your forearm against the floor to raise your hips until your body is straight from your ankles to your shoulders. Hold the bridge for 15 to 45 seconds, then repeat the exercise on your left side. Remember to contract your abs and butt muscles forcefully to keep your body straight.

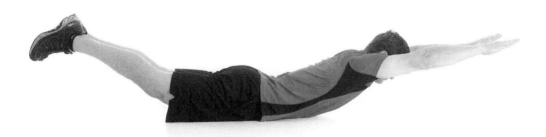

SUPERMAN (LOWER BACK)

Lie facedown and extend your arms in front of you. Tightening your lower back, simultaneously raise your arms and legs off the floor. Hold for 2 seconds, then release, and repeat.

ADDITIONAL CORE EXERCISES

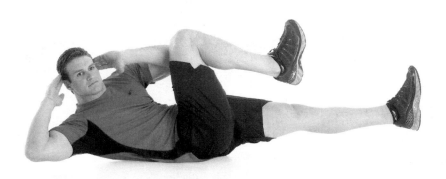

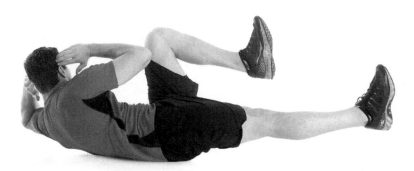

BICYCLE (UPPER AND LOWER ABS)

When researchers at the Biomechanics Lab at San Diego State University measured muscle stimulation of subjects doing different abs exercises, they found that the bicycle crunch engaged more abs muscles than any of 12 other exercises. How to do it right: Lie on your back with your knees bent 90 degrees and your fingertips lightly touching your ears. Pump your legs back and forth, bicycle style, while rotating your torso from side to side. You should try to point your armpit, instead of your elbow, toward the opposite knee on each pump. That'll accentuate your torso rotation. Breathe evenly throughout the exercise.

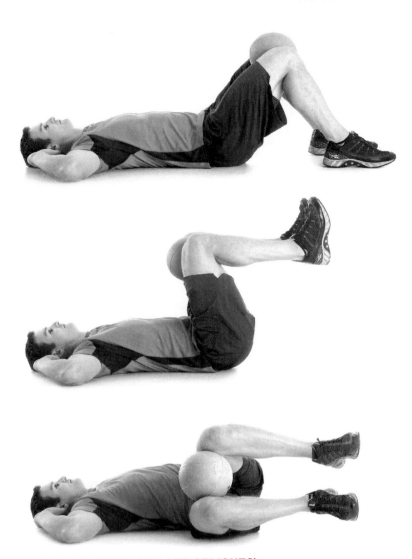

KNEE RAISE WITH DROP (LOWER ABS AND OBLIQUES)

Lie on your back and squeeze a medicine ball between your bent knees. Put your hands behind your ears and place your feet flat on the floor. Contract your abdominals while pulling your knees to your chest and your feet off the floor. Next, lower your knees to the right, bring them back to the center, then return to the starting position. Now pull your knees to your chest again, drop them to the left this time, and bring them back to the center. That's 1 rep. Continue alternating sides.

ADDITIONAL CORE EXERCISES

SUPERSHOT
Hang in There

Boost your endurance with this challenge: Do as many hanging knee raises as you can, then rest for 30 seconds. Repeat three times. That counts as 1 set. Do 2 or 3 sets—resting for 60 to 90 seconds after each—two or three times a week. Each week, shorten your within-set rest by 5 seconds until you can do 10 reps straight.

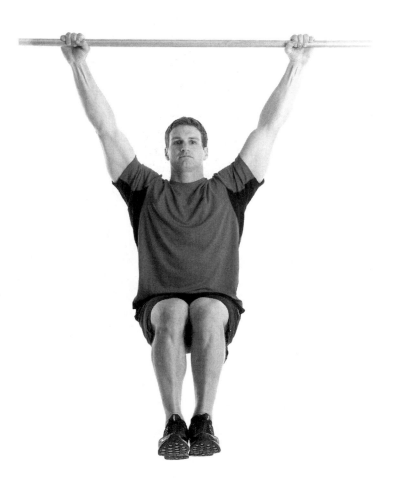

HANGING KNEE RAISE (LOWER ABS)

Hang with your arms extended straight from a chinup bar. Your palms are facing out and hands a bit past shoulder-width apart. Raise your knees toward your chest, curling your pelvis upward at the end.

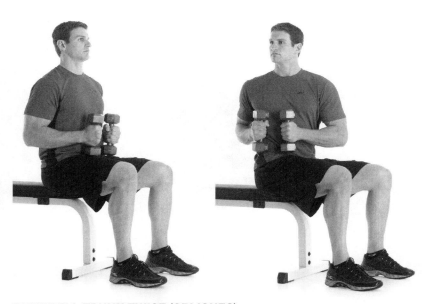

DUMBBELL TRUNK TWIST (OBLIQUES)

Sit at the edge of a bench with your feet flat on the floor. Keep your chest out and your head aligned with your torso. Hold a light dumbbell in each hand, palms facing your body. Bend your arms and bring the weights close to your belly. Now, slowly and smoothly twist your torso to the right as far as you can comfortably go. Hold this spot for a second, then slowly return to the starting position. Repeat the move to the left, then continue alternating right and left until your muscles are fatigued.

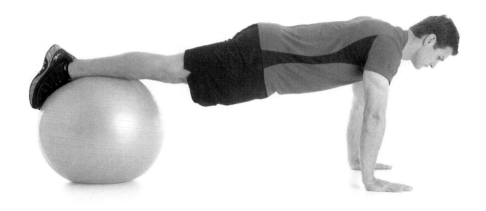

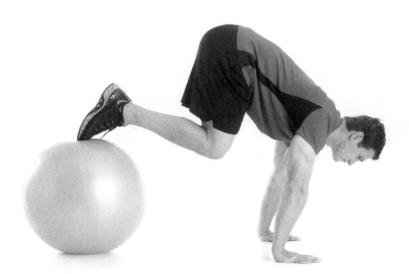

STABILITY BALL KNEE TUCK (TRANSVERSE ABDOMINIS)
Get into a pushup position with your shins resting on a stability ball
and your hands slightly more than shoulder-width apart. Keeping
your abs tight, lift your hips and draw your knees toward your chest
until your shins rise off the ball and your toes are on top of the ball.
Slowly straighten your legs so that the ball rolls back to the starting
position.

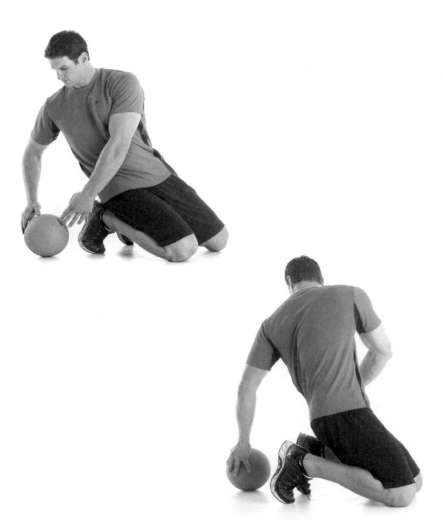

MEDICINE BALL TORSO ROTATION (OBLIQUES)

Kneel down with your feet on the floor behind you. Hold a medicine ball or basketball in front of you. Quickly twist to your right, and set the ball down behind your back. Twist to the left, and pick up the ball. Bring the ball around to your right, and set it down again. Repeat. After completing a set this way, do the same number of repetitions this time twisting first to the left.

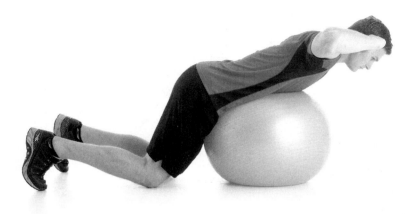

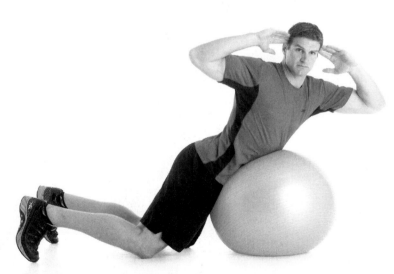

TWISTING BACK EXTENSION (LOWER BACK)

Lie facedown on a stability ball so that your waist rests on the ball and your legs hang off with your feet touching the ground as shown. (If you have a partner, ask him or her to hold your ankles down.) Place your hands so that your fingers are lightly touching your ears. Lower your upper body, allowing your lower back to round around the ball, then raise your torso until it's slightly above parallel to the floor; this is the starting position. Now twist your upper body to the right. Pause, then lower your torso to the starting position and twist to the left. Pause, then return to the starting position again. That's 1 repetition.

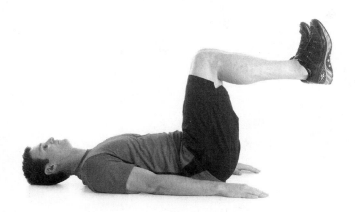

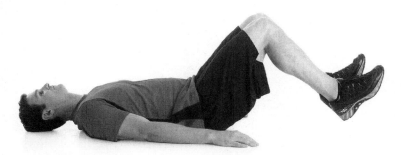

FLAT BACK LEG-LOWERING DRILL (ABS AND HIP FLEXORS)

Lie on your back and raise your legs over your hips, with your knees slightly bent. Press the small of your back into the floor to eliminate the arch in your lower back. Keep your back in this position as you take 3 to 5 seconds to lower your legs. Upon reaching the lowest point at which you can still keep your back flat, bring your legs to your chest. Try to lower your legs more with each repetition.

REAL GUYS—REAL RESULTS

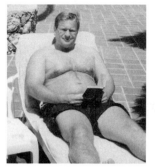

BEFORE:
250
POUNDS

AFTER:
180
POUNDS

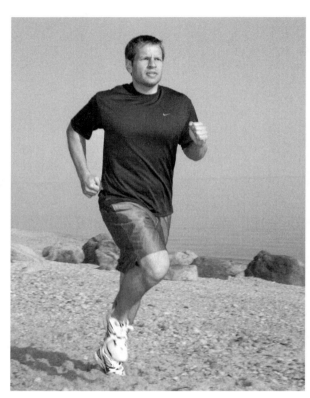

"I finally have the energy to play with my kids."

VITALS: **Chris Williams, 32, Wading River, NY**
OCCUPATION: **Teacher**
HEIGHT: **5'10"**
LESSON LEARNED: **Expect roadblocks; beating them gave me encouragement.**

Williams grew up on cookies, cakes, and other foods loaded with junk carbohydrates. He was forced to start his first diet at age 11. But it didn't work. By the time he got married, he had ballooned to 250 pounds.

THE TURNING POINT

His wife became pregnant. "I knew something would have to change once my daughter was born," Williams says, "so I could run around with her and not wipe myself out."

LIFE IN THE FIT LANE

Williams combines running and biking with circuit training. "It wasn't too difficult to start working out, but once I started to eat right, it became even easier." Williams follows a protein-rich diet, filling his plate with chicken, turkey, and lean beef and supplementing with whole grains and veg-etables. He boosted his cardio workouts to 60 minutes, 5 days a week, and lifts weights 4 days a week. Now he runs 10-Ks and recently completed a triathlon. He even became a part-time personal trainer, something he always wanted to do, but never had the energy to pursue.

THE REWARD

Beyond the satisfaction of trimming his body fat down to an amazing 7 percent, Williams is able to keep up with his kids without losing his breath. And his wife and children are encouraged to follow his example of healthy eating. "Maintaining my weight has given me a huge sense of accomplishment," he says.

WILLIAMS'S BEST BELLY OFF! TIPS

● Shun fads. Losing weight is truly a simple balance of a low-calorie diet coupled with exercise.
● Don't feel guilty. On days when you miss a workout or eat too much, chalk it up to being human. Give yourself a break.
● Keep a photograph of yourself at your heaviest for motivation.

11

FAST FITNESS
15-Minute Workouts That'll Bust Your Gut

OW MANY TIMES have you thought, "I just don't have time to exercise"?

Lack of time is the number one reason people say that they have difficulty sticking with a fitness program. Time. It's one of our most precious personal commodities. Other priorities—work, eating, family, socializing, watching YouTube, did I mention work?—take precedence over exercise time. But you know that.

So what if working out took just a little bit of time? Say, 15 minutes? Could you find 15 minutes to squeeze in something so vital to your life, so vital to the way you look and feel and the way you perform during the rest of your day?

In 24 hours there are 96 individual 15-minute segments—64, if you subtract the time you spend asleep. That's 64 opportunities to fit exercise into your day. The average American spends 2.6 hours a day watching television. That's 10 possibilities right there.

The average American spends 1.5 hours surfing the Web every day—another 6 opportunities to sweat.

Finding the 15 isn't hard. *Doing the 15*—that's the tough part. Taking that first step out of your street clothes and into your jockstrap. Lacing up your running shoes. Getting moving. All of that is up to you. Nobody is going to take you by the hand. But it helps to have a plan. So here is yours. In this chapter, you'll find 13 different workouts, most designed to take no longer than 15 minutes. They are brief, but that doesn't mean they are easy. In fact, because you do them so quickly, some of them may have you vomiting in the bushes. But that's okay. Wipe off your shoes. Exercise perfect form, push yourself hard, and you will experience total-body, belly-busting pumps that'll rival most workouts that take an hour or longer. Your 15 minutes starts . . . *now*.

ANYWHERE, MINIMAL-GEAR WORKOUTS

WORKOUT 1: HOTEL ROOM BODYWEIGHT CIRCUIT

Complete this circuit twice without resting.

EXERCISE	REPS
Plank	30 seconds in position 1 30 seconds in position 2
Partial Split Squat	10 reps per side
T-Pushup	10-20 reps
Stepup	10-20 reps per side

WORKOUT **1**

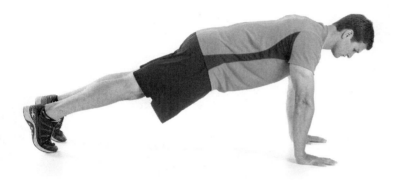

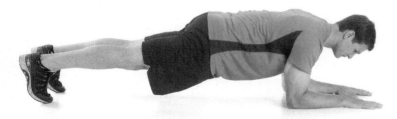

PLANK

Get into pushup position with your ankles, knees, hips, back, and head in a straight line. Hold the pose for 30 seconds while tightening your abs. Next, bend your elbows so that you support your body with your forearms on the floor. Hold this position for 30 seconds.

WORKOUT **1**

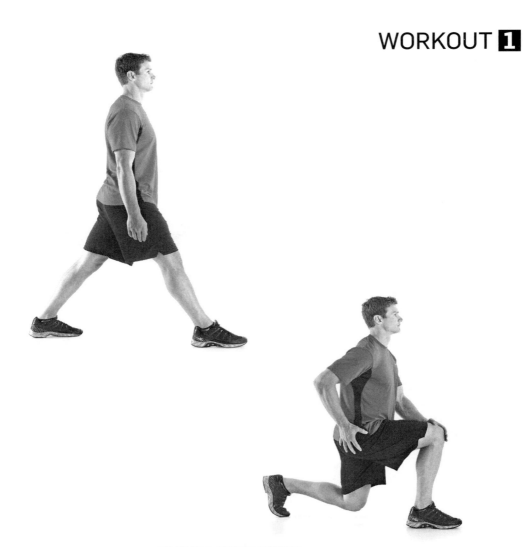

PARTIAL SPLIT SQUAT

Step forward with your right leg, taking a bigger-than-normal step. Keep your upper body upright and your arms at your sides. Bend your right leg to 90 degrees, keeping your right knee in line with your ankle. Lower your left leg until your knee touches the floor. Place your left hand on the inside of your right knee and put your right hand on your right butt muscle. Raise your left knee 1 inch off the floor. This is the starting position. Raise yourself by extending both legs; you'll feel tension in your knee and butt. Pause, then return to the starting position, with your left knee 1 inch off the floor. Complete 10 reps, then switch legs and repeat.

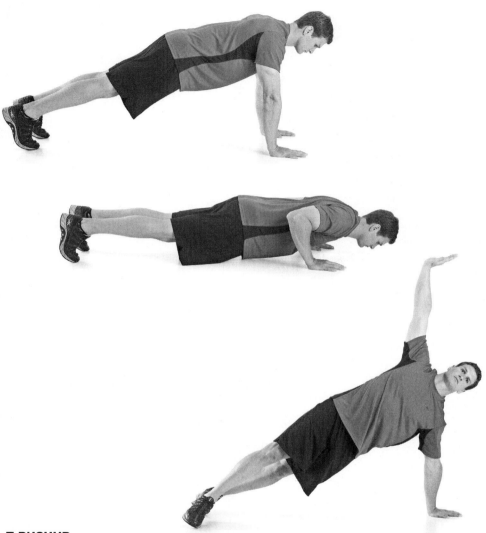

T-PUSHUP

Get into normal pushup position. Lower yourself and then push yourself up. When you reach the top, elbows-locked position, transfer you bodyweight to your left arm and rotate your body to the right. Reach up and behind you with your right arm. Your feet will rotate as well. Hold for 2 seconds. (You can make this move harder by lifting your right foot off the floor at the end of the movement to make an X shape with your arms and legs.) Return to the starting position and repeat on the other side with your left arm raised. Perform 10 to 20 repetitions.

WORKOUT **1**

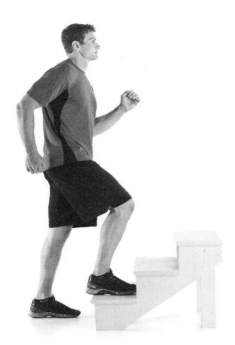

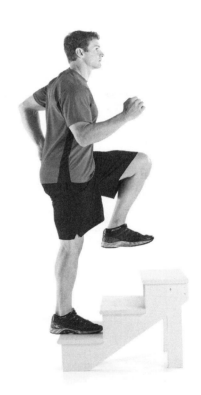

STEPUP

Stand facing a staircase, and place your right foot on the bottom step. Using only your right leg, push yourself up until you can straighten that leg, then lift your left knee as shown. Slowly lower yourself, keeping your right foot on the step. Lower your left leg to return to the starting position. Repeat 10 to 20 times. Then place your left foot on the step to repeat the exercise on the right side.

WORKOUT 2: QUICK STEPS

This workout combines cardiovascular drills with strength exercises to build muscle and burn calories. All you need is a staircase or a bench. Alternate between the sprinter's step drill and elevated feet pushup for 2 sets before moving on to the upper-body shuttle.

EXERCISE	REPS
Sprinter's Step Drill	30 seconds
Elevated Feet Pushup	10-15 reps
Sprinter's Step Drill	30 seconds
Elevated Feet Pushup	10-15 reps
Upper-Body Shuttle	30-60 seconds

WORKOUT **2**

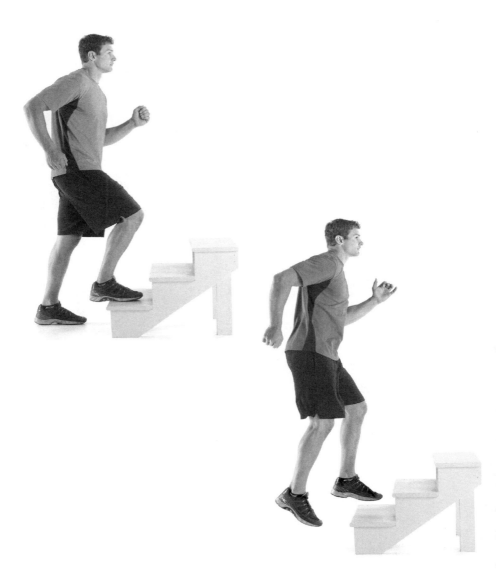

SPRINTER'S STEP DRILL

Stand facing a bench or stair step with your right foot on the step and your right knee bent. Rapidly alternate your feet on and off the step so you're sprinting in place. Drive your knees up and pump your arms as if you were sprinting. Continue for 30 seconds.

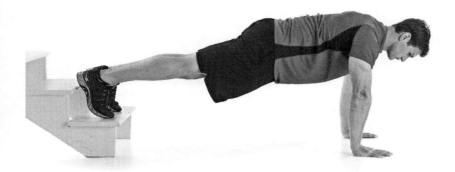

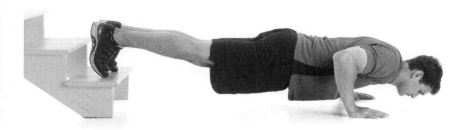

ELEVATED-FEET PUSHUP

Get into the pushup position, facing away from the stairs, with the
balls of your feet on the bottom step. Brace your abs and keep your
back flat. Bend your elbows and lower yourself until your chest is a
couple of inches off the floor. Pause, then push back up. Do 10 to
15 repetitions.

DADDY-DUTY DRILLS

How Pops Can Get a T-shirt-Drenching Workout at the Playground

I have a 2$\frac{1}{2}$-year-old named Sophia. Sophia likes to go to the playground. I don't like to go to the playground. But Sophia likes the playground.

So we go to the playground.

"Daddy, I swing? Daddy, I swing? Daddy, I swing? Daddy, I swing?" Believe me, it's far better to go to the playground right away than to listen to that for 23 minutes, and then give in.

It didn't take my multitasking mind long to figure out that while Sophia swings, Daddy could get in a workout using all the neat apparatuses at the playground. I mean, hell, it's called the Jungle Gym after all. There are bars for pullups, steps for stepups, rings and swings for dips and elevated pushups. If you can't put together a couple of good circuits on all that stuff, well, you're just not tapping your inner kid.

And lest you think that you're doing a disservice to your child by not spending "quality time" with him or her, let me set your mind straight: Get over it. Who cares what the moms chatting on the bench think? Are they doing any better gossiping about Mary's affair with her chiropractor?

Sophia thinks I'm playing right along with her. And really getting into it. I can tell by her smiles and squeals. She loves going to the playground with Daddy. And now Daddy loves it, too.

Here's the circuit I did the other day, though the order of exercises changes each time we visit, depending upon which swing or slide or other equipment she wants to climb upon. Do the circuit two or three times with a 5-minute rest between circuits. You'll leave the park with a happy child and a total-body pump. By the way, anyone can do this workout—you don't need a child for motivation. This is a bodyweight workout for everyone who's a child at heart.

Reverse Crunch on a Swing. Get on the ground in front of a swing as if you were about to do a pushup—placing your hands shoulder-width apart. But instead of straightening your legs with your feet on the ground, place them on a swing so the fronts of your shins rest on the seat. You've done this move on a stability ball. Here, instead of the ball rolling, you've got a swing swinging. With your arms straight and your back flat, slowly bend your legs and bring the swing seat toward your chest, raising your hips, tightening your abs, and rounding your back as you go. Pause, return to the starting position, and repeat.

Slide Incline Pushup. Get into a pushup position and place your feet on the second rung of the slide ladder or convenient stair steps. Straighten your body, then lower yourself until your upper arms are parallel to the ground, then press yourself back up and repeat.

Knee Raise on the Monkey Bars. Hang from the monkey bars with your arms slightly wider than shoulder-width apart, your palms facing forward, and knees bent with your feet behind you. Keeping your feet together, slowly raise them to your chest. Pause for 2 seconds, then slowly lower them, and repeat. Other monkey-bar moves: chinups, pullups, and dips.

Park Bench Jackknife Pushup. Sometimes called a handstand pushup, the jackknife targets your shoulders and forces your core to stabilize your body during the movement. Place your feet on a park bench or step and your hands on the ground in the pushup position. Now walk your hands back toward your feet until your body forms an inverted V and your upper body is nearly vertical. Lower your body by bending your arms until your head nears the ground, then drive back up to the starting position by straightening your arms.

Stair Stepup. Find a park bench or a high stair step. Stand in front of it. Place your right foot on the bench. Pressing your heel into the step, stand up using only the power of that leg. Slowly, under control, lower yourself to the starting position and repeat 10 times. Then do the same exercise with your left leg.

Horizontal Pullup. Find a horizontal bar that's about 3 feet off the ground, high enough to hang straight-armed underneath without your back touching the ground. (Look around on the jungle gym or those fancy "forts" that we never had when we were kids.) Your hands should be shoulder-width apart on the bar. Your legs will be extended in front of you and your body stiff and tight. Pull up until your chest touches the bar (slightly above nipple line) and lower until your arms are completely extended. Do a set of 10, then turn your palms up and take a narrow grip on the bar (hands about a foot apart). Do another 10 reps this way.

Piggyback Walking Lunge. Give your kid a piggyback ride. Tell him or her to hold on to your neck tightly. Now, do walking lunges. To avoid injury (to you), make sure your forward knee doesn't travel out in front of your toes. A set of 20, done slowly, with the added weight on your back, will give you a heart-pounding workout. And your kid will love the up-and-down ride.

Sophia Squat Press. I grab my daughter under her armpits so she's facing me and I bring her to my chest. From that position, I do a full squat. After straightening my legs, I lift her above my head as if doing a dumbbell press with my palms facing each other. She loves that part. That's 1 rep. I do 8, then we rest. Sophia always says, "Again?"

WORKOUT 2

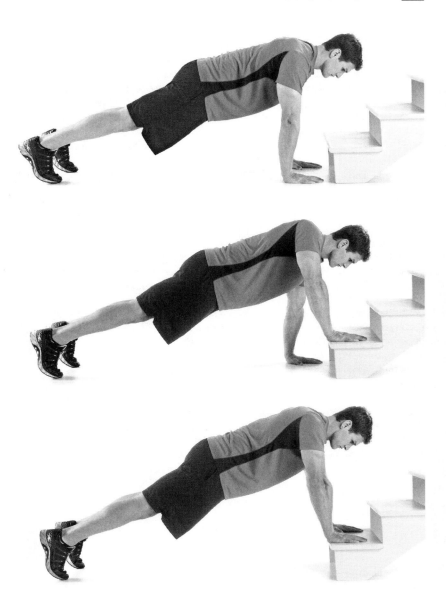

UPPER-BODY SHUTTLE

Face the stairs in a pushup position, with your fingertips just in front of the bottom step. Lift one hand onto the step, then bring up your other hand. Return your first hand to the floor, then the second. Walk your hands up and down this way for 30 to 60 seconds.

WORKOUT 3: MEDICINE BALL LADDER

This grueling four-drill circuit incinerates belly fat. Incorporating a medicine ball adds interest, difficulty, and an upper-body element. Do each of the exercises for 30 seconds, then rest for 1 minute. Repeat the circuit, this time performing each move for 45 seconds. Rest for 90 seconds, then repeat once more, doing each move for 60 seconds.

EXERCISE	TIME
Side-to-Side Shuffle	30 seconds
Overhead Lunge Walk	30 seconds
Medicine Ball 180	30 seconds
Pushup Shuttle	30 seconds
REST	1 minute
Side-to-Side Shuffle	45 seconds
Overhead Lunge Walk	45 seconds
Medicine Ball 180	45 seconds
Pushup Shuttle	45 seconds
REST	90 seconds
Side-to-Side Shuffle	60 seconds
Overhead Lunge Walk	60 seconds
Medicine Ball 180	60 seconds
Pushup Shuttle	60 seconds

FIT FACT

40

Percentage reduction in risk of disability and death from all major diseases that middle-aged and older runners can expect by running regularly, according to a 21-year study of 440 runners and healthy nonrunners by Stanford University researchers

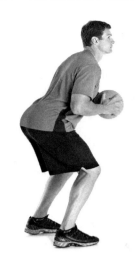

WORKOUT 3

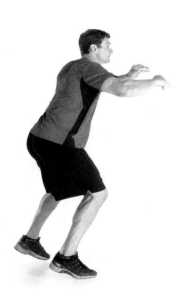

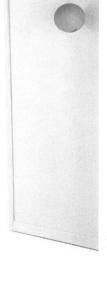

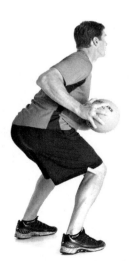

SIDE-TO-SIDE SHUFFLE

Stand facing a wall from 5 feet away, holding a medicine ball at chest height. Throw the ball at the wall 3 to 5 feet to your right and at eye level. As the ball bounces off the wall, shuffle sideways and catch it on a bounce before firing it back to your left.

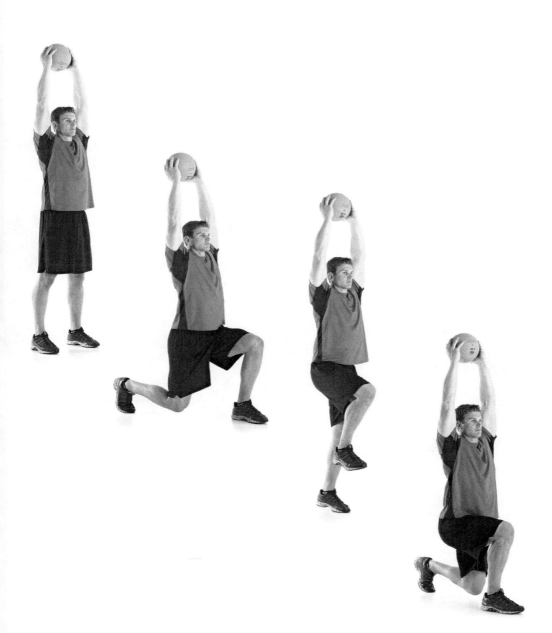

OVERHEAD LUNGE WALK

Stand holding a medicine ball overhead at arm's length. Keeping your arms straight, take a large step forward until both knees are bent 90 degrees and your back knee is an inch or two off the floor. Stride forward with the opposite leg.

WORKOUT 3

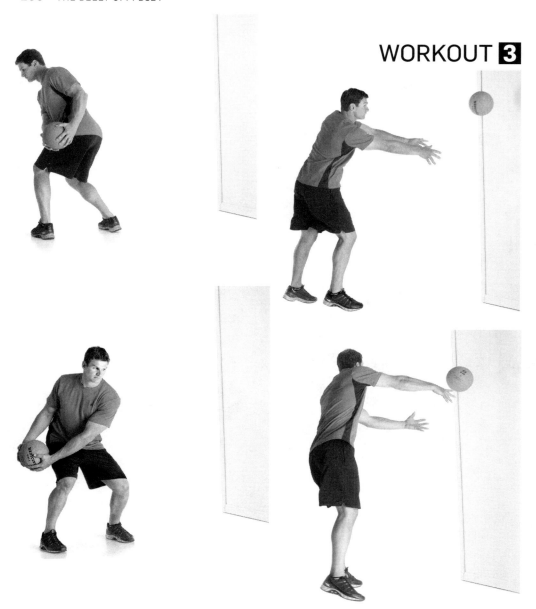

MEDICINE BALL 180

Stand about 5 feet away from a wall so that the right side of your body is facing the wall. Hold a medicine ball in front of your chest, arms straight. Rotate your torso away from the wall slightly, then rotate forcefully toward the wall, throwing the ball at the wall and slightly behind you. Turn around and shuffle over to catch the ball on a bounce, then face the left side of your body toward the wall and repeat the move in the opposite direction.

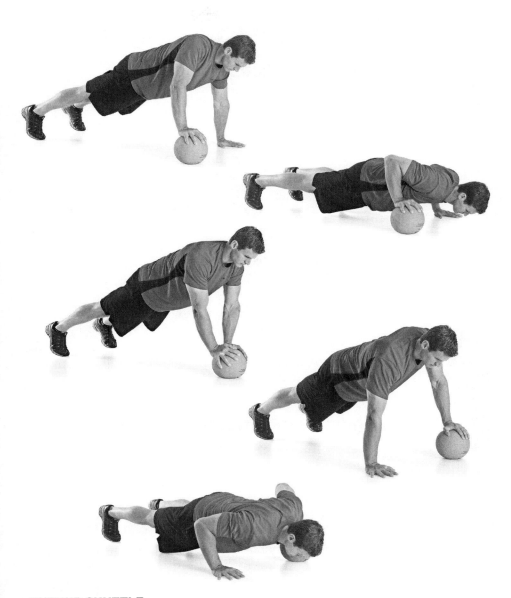

PUSHUP SHUTTLE

Assume the classic pushup position, but instead of placing both hands on the floor, place your right hand on a medicine ball. Bend your arms to lower your body toward the floor. Push yourself up, then transfer your left hand to the medicine ball. Next, move your right hand to the floor to perform a pushup.

CHALLENGING INTERVALS

WORKOUT 4: GRANDSTANDS

Go to a high school football stadium and run grandstand repeats.

- Sprint to the top of the stands at 80 to 90 percent effort, turn around, then walk or jog back down. Repeat 10 times.

- Rest for 60 seconds, then do 10 more sprints to the top.

- Rest for 90 seconds.

- For your final set, sprint up four steps, turn around and jog back down. Then sprint five steps, turn around and jog back down. Continue this way, six steps; turn around; seven, turn around, and so on until you reach the top step.

WORKOUT 5: ROWING FAT-BURNER

Irish researchers recently reported that men burn 40 to 50 percent more fat when rowing than when cycling. That's because rowing machines require equal effort from both your upper and lower body. But proper technique is key. On the back stroke, your knees should be almost completely straight before you squeeze your shoulder blades together and pull the handle to your sternum. You should maintain a curve in your lower back during the entire movement.

- Start with a 5-minute warmup of easy rowing.

- Do a set of 10 power strokes, where you pull the handle to your torso as fast and as hard as you can, then slow down to half effort for 60 seconds.

- Perform 15 power strokes at maximum effort, then slow down to half effort for 60 seconds.

- Do 20 power strokes followed by 60 seconds of easy rowing. Repeat this cycle for 10 minutes.

LEARN THE ROPES TO LOSE MORE WEIGHT
Jumping Rope Will Help You Skip Big Meals

A jump rope is one of the cheapest yet most effective pieces of exercise equipment. If you don't have one, put down this book and go get one. Just 10 minutes of jumping rope can provide the same calorie burn as 30 minutes of running. It'll enhance your performance in basketball, tennis, skiing, soccer, volleyball, and other jumping sports. Plus, when you get good enough to do those front crosses and single side swings, you'll look like a prize-fighter—featherweight, of course.

Rope jumping takes a bit of coordination and practice because it uses all your muscles and joints. Here are some pointers.

How to balance: Keep your weight on the balls of your feet. Bend your knees slightly. The trick is to keep your jumps shallow; don't jump more than an inch. Keep your body upright and your elbows close to your sides. Make small circles with your wrists.

How to jump: It's just a slight push, coming from the movement of your ankles, calves, knees, and hips. Push through the floor with the balls of your feet and point your toes downward as you lift off.

How to land: Land softly by spreading the impact through your ankles, knees, and hips. Don't think too hard about it. Just keep your heels from touching the ground and you'll do fine.

Try the alternate step: Jump with one foot. On the second turn of the rope, switch feet. Continue alternating your feet as if jogging in place at a comfortable rhythm. Lift your knees forward without kicking backward, which can cause your foot to catch on the rope.

The workout: Using the basic bounce or alternate step, start with 10 sets of 10 jumps. Increase the number of jumps by 10 per set until you reach 100 jumps nonstop.

Once you become proficient, try this jump rope interval workout:

ADVANCED INTERVAL

Pack a jump rope in your suitcase on your next business trip. Jumping rope for just 15 minutes will give you an unparalleled total-body workout. Warm up with 5 minutes of easy skipping.
- Increase your speed to 80 percent of your maximum effort for 30 seconds.
- Skip easily for 60 seconds.
- Do high-knee skips for 30 seconds.
- Skip easily for 60 seconds.
- Continue this pattern for two more cycles.
- For the last 5 minutes, alternate between skipping as fast as you can for 60 seconds and easy skipping for 60 seconds.

WORKOUT 6:
KNEE-SAVING ELLIPTICAL INTERVAL

To boost the cardiovascular benefits and burn more calories, don't hold the handles. Instead, pump your arms as if you were running.

- After a 5-minute warmup of easy striding, increase the machine's resistance level until you're working at 80 percent of your maximum effort. Keep this up for 2 minutes.

- Next, lower the resistance to the level you started with for your warmup, but quicken your stride so that you're still exercising at 80 percent of your full effort. Continue for 2 minutes.

- Alternate between high resistance and fast stride every 2 minutes for a total of 10 minutes.

WORKOUT 7:
EASY RUNNING INTERVAL OUTDOORS

The following workout is an excellent step toward building the stamina for high-intensity interval training.

WARMUP: 5 MINUTES OF EASY JOGGING

Sprint	Recovery (60 percent of maximum effort)
30 seconds	90 seconds
30 seconds	90 seconds
30 seconds	90 seconds
30 seconds	90 seconds

COOLDOWN: 3 MINUTES OF EASY JOGGING

WORKOUT 8:
TOUGH RUNNING INTERVAL OUTDOORS

WARMUP: 5 MINUTES OF EASY JOGGING

Sprint	Recovery (60 percent of maximum effort)
30 seconds	30 seconds
25 seconds	30 seconds
25 seconds	30 seconds
20 seconds	30 seconds
20 seconds	30 seconds
15 seconds	30 seconds
15 seconds	30 seconds

COOLDOWN: 5 MINUTES OF EASY JOGGING

WORKOUT 9: UP-THE-INCLINE TREADMILL INTERVAL (20 MINUTES)

To mimic road running, raise the incline of the treadmill to 1 percent before starting your run. Researchers have found that 1 degree of treadmill elevation closely approximates outdoor running.

Punch in a treadmill speed of moderate intensity, one that allows you to carry on a conversation while running. Run at that speed for 2 minutes, then raise the incline to 4 percent. Continue raising the elevation of the treadmill by 2 percent every 2 minutes until you reach a 10 percent grade. Then step it back 1 percent at a time in 1-minute intervals.

WORKOUT 10: STEP-DOWN FARTLEK (30 TO 40 MINUTES)

Fartlek is Swedish for "speed play," meaning you accelerate and slow down according to how you feel. I love to do 30-minute fartlek runs in my neighborhood. I start out running at an easy clip for 5 minutes to warm up. Then I'll sprint as hard as I can for as long as I can before slowing down to an easy jog to catch my breath. Then I'll repeat the sequence. Or

SUPERSHOT
Gain Power with a Shrug

Load a barbell and roll it to your shins. Squat down and grab it with an overhand grip. In one explosive motion, pull the bar off the floor, straighten your legs, rise onto your toes, and shrug your shoulders. Then lower the bar to the floor. (Keep your arms straight down as you shrug your shoulders.)

catch my breath. Then I'll repeat the sequence. Or sometimes I'll choose two points ahead of me on my route, a telephone pole, for example, and a mailbox 50 to 100 yards ahead. Once I pass the telephone pole, I'll sprint to the mailbox, then slow down again to a speed that's about 40 percent of my maximum sprint speed. I'll recover at this pace, then look for another set of landmarks that catches my fancy to sprint between.

In a "step-down fartlek," you put your feelings aside and follow a set structure. These intervals become harder at the end of your run, mimicking how you would feel at the end of a race.

Start at a pace that's about 60 percent of your full effort and go for 5 minutes. Then slow down to about 40 percent effort for 5 minutes. Next increase speed to about 70 percent of your full effort and go for 4 minutes. Continue this fast-then-slow pattern, but shorten the hard-running segment by a minute each time while increasing your speed slightly. By the last 1-minute burst, you should be almost sprinting.

AT-HOME OR IN-GYM WEIGHT WORKOUTS

WORKOUT 11: PUSH-PULL WITH DUMBBELLS AND BARBELLS

Do 2 to 3 sets of 8 to 10 repetitions of each exercise before moving on to the next. Rest 30 seconds between sets.

EXERCISE	REPS
Dumbbell Bulgarian Split-Squat Press	8-10 reps
Dumbbell Squat Press	8-10 reps
Dumbbell One-Arm Bench Press on Stability Ball	8-10 reps on each side
Bent-over Row and Romanian Deadlift	8-10 reps

WORKOUT **11**

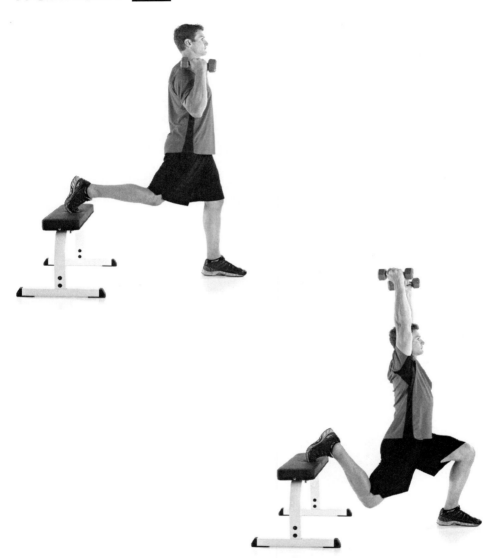

DUMBBELL BULGARIAN SPLIT-SQUAT PRESS

Bend your right knee and place your right foot on a bench behind you.
Hold a pair of light dumbbells at your shoulders. As you descend into
a squat, simultaneously press the dumbbells overhead. As you
straighten your left leg, bring the weights back to your shoulders. Do
8 to 10 repetitions, then switch legs, performing the same number of
reps with your left foot on the bench.

WORKOUT **11**

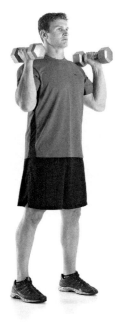

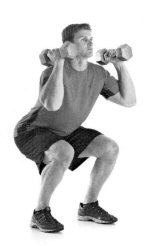

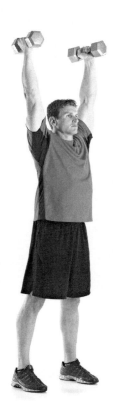

DUMBBELL SQUAT PRESS

Stand with feet shoulder-width apart and dumbbells resting on your shoulders. Descend into a deep squat and drive the weights overhead as you rise from the bottom of the squat.

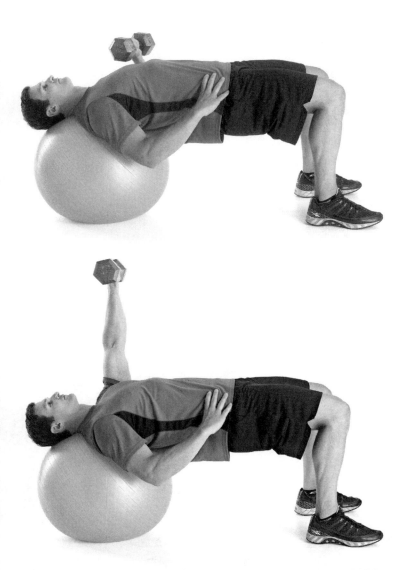

DUMBBELL ONE-ARM BENCH PRESS ON STABILITY BALL

Lie with your upper back on a stability ball and hold a dumbbell in
your left hand. (Place your right hand on your hip.) Hold the weight at
your chest and perform a one-arm bench press. Do 8 to 10 reps, then
transfer the weight to your right hand and repeat the same number
of reps.

WORKOUT 11

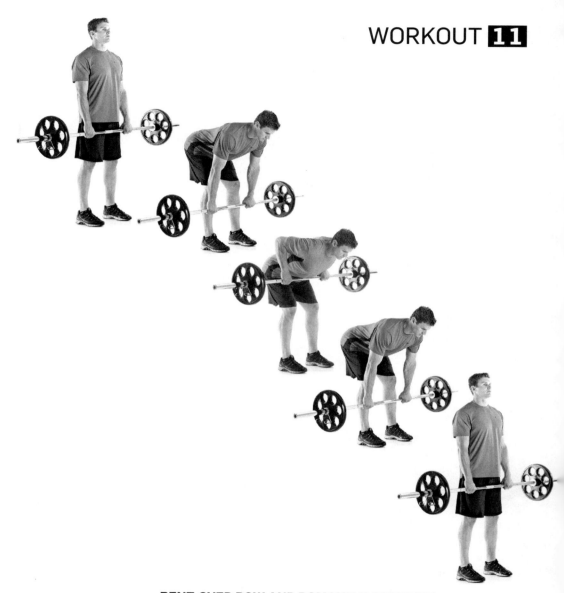

BENT-OVER ROW AND ROMANIAN DEADLIFT

Stand with your feet shoulder-width apart, with your hands grasping a barbell in an overhand grip slightly wider than shoulder width. Now bend at the waist until your lower back is flat; bend your knees slightly. Row the weight up until the bar makes contact with your lower rib cage. Lower the bar until your arms are completely extended. At this point, do a deadlift (see page 140). Then repeat the two-lift sequence 8 to 10 times.

WORKOUT 12: THE STOP-AND-GO SUPERSETS

The Stop-and-Go is a terrific plateau-busting work-out. By interrupting momentum at various power points, you recruit more muscle fibers, making each rep tougher. The result: more calories burned and more strength at your weak spots.

The plan: Do the pushups and split squats without resting between exercises. Then rest for 30 seconds and repeat the superset. Next, do the dumbbell row and the sumo squat as another superset.

EXERCISE	REPS
Superset 1	
Stop-and-Go Pushup	8 reps
Stop-and-Go Split Squat	8 reps
REST	30 seconds
Superset 2	
Stop-and-Go Incline Dumbbell Row	10 reps
Stop-and-Go Sumo Squat	10 reps

WORKOUT 12

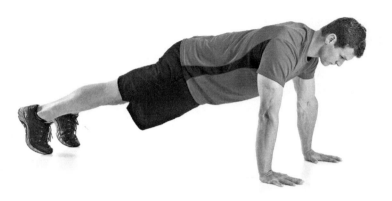

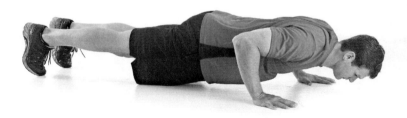

SUPERSET 1

STOP-AND-GO PUSHUP

Assume a pushup position. Brace your core and lower your chest to the floor. When you're halfway down, pause for 2 seconds before continuing. Then, when your chest is 2 inches from the floor, pause again for 2 seconds before pushing halfway back up. Hold for 2 more seconds, then straighten your arms. Do 8 reps.

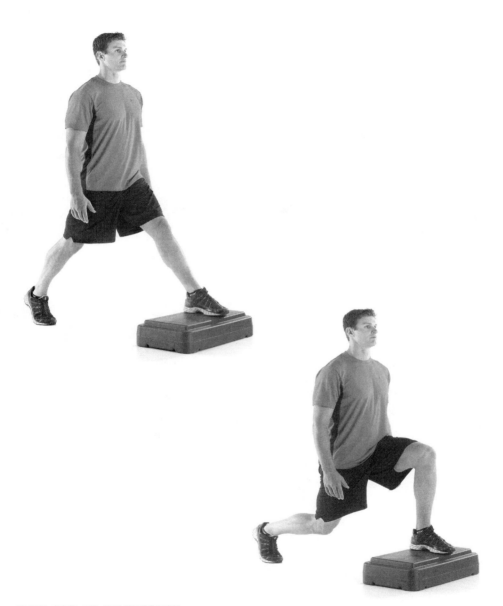

STOP-AND-GO SPLIT SQUAT

Stand with one foot 3 feet forward on a step. Rise on the ball of your
back foot, then bend at the knees. When halfway down, pause for
2 seconds. Pause again when your back knee is just off the floor.
Push halfway up, pause again, and return to the starting position.
Do 8 reps with each leg.

WORKOUT 12

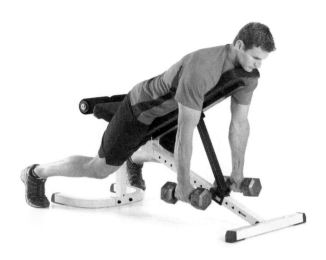

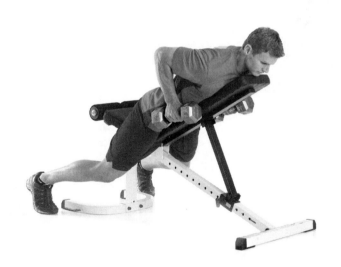

SUPERSET 2

STOP-AND-GO INCLINE DUMBBELL ROW

Holding dumbbells, lie face down on a bench set at 45 degrees. Pull the dumbbells up toward your torso. When your upper arms align with your torso, pause 2 seconds before continuing, until the dumbbells are at your sides. Hold for two beats, then lower halfway and pause again. Return to the starting position. Do 10 reps.

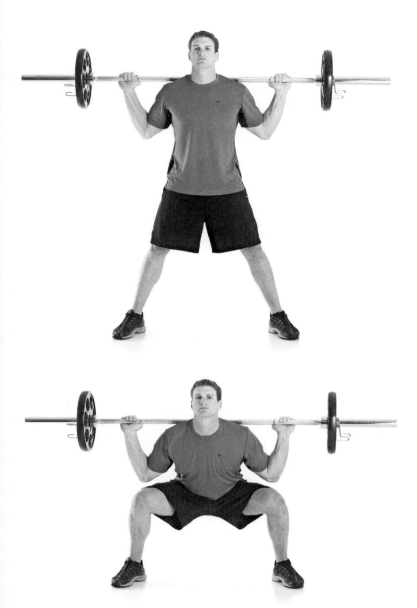

STOP-AND-GO SUMO SQUAT

Stand holding a barbell across your shoulders, feet wide apart with toes turned out. Bend at the knees to lower your body. Halfway down, pause 2 seconds before continuing until your thighs are parallel to the floor. Pause two beats, then press halfway up and pause again before returning to the starting position. Do 10 reps.

WORKOUT 13: THE TWO-SET CLASSIC

Rest 30 seconds between sets.

Squat	
Set 1	8 to 12 reps
Set 2	6 to 8 reps
Deadlift (page 140)	
Set 1	8 to 12 reps
Set 2	6 to 8 reps
Forward Lunge (page 86)	
Set 1	8 to 12 reps
Set 2	6 to 8 reps
Dumbbell Bench Press (page 119)	
Set 1	8 to 12 reps
Set 2	6 to 8 reps
Bent-Over Row (page 296)	
Set 1	8 to 12 reps
Set 2	6 to 8 reps
Seated Dumbbell Shoulder Press (page 120)	
Set 1	8 to 12 reps
Set 2	6 to 8 reps
Biceps Curl (page 121)	
Set 1	8 to 12 reps
Set 2	6 to 8 reps
Crunch (page 123)	
1 set (done until failure)	

12

TRAVELING LIGHT

Don't Get Saddled with Extra
Baggage on Business Trips

W ELCOME TO THE BUSINESS TRIP of
your dreams: You can arrive at the
airport an hour before your flight.
There's no body cavity search at
the security check, and you are
free to leave your shoes on. The
plane isn't crowded. The seats are leather and roomy.
Your neighbor is pretty, friendly, and interesting. Your
bags arrive with you.

And you won't put on 5 pounds by the time you get
back home.

Now wake up, pal. Bring your seatback and tray
table up and put away all unapproved electronic
devices. The reality of business travel is that it can
easily knock you out of your fitness routine and botch
up your best intentions to eat healthfully. You've
been there. You've learned that there's no glamour in
business travel after your second layover in Dubuque
or Dubai.

But you have to do it. Because making it happen at work often means getting *out there* to make it happen. And, besides, the boss says you have to go.

There are right ways to travel to minimize the toll it takes on your body and there are wrong ways. The problem with business trips is that people turn it into a special event that allows them to break sound nutrition rules, says Susan Bowerman, a registered dietitian and assistant director for the UCLA Center for Human Nutrition.

Isn't that the truth? Not long ago, I got on a business-class flight to Milan, Italy. Here's how it went: I sipped the pre-takeoff champagne. I ate the warm salted nuts. Two little bowls. I had a beer. When dinner arrived, I tried the wine, the chardonnay. I went for the cheese plate after dinner with a glass of Barolo. A little later, the ice cream sundae. A bit of cognac while watching the movies. Then . . . *breakfast!* Mimosas?!

By the time I arrived at Malpensa Airport, I was bleary eyed and covered in crumbs. And I felt like *merda*. Until I had a double espresso. There was espresso at every meeting. And tasty little pastries. We ate big lunches with wine. I remember with particular admiration a *cotoletta alla Milanese* at a perfect old farmhouse restaurant in Segrate. The breaded and fried veal cutlet was the size of a personal pan pizza. And speaking of pizza, we had many kinds that night with more wine. I love Italy. And it loves me back. *Grazie!* I return home with many souvenirs tucked under my belt.

After a couple of those trips to Italy, I decided that my 18-hour flight to Cape Town, South Africa, would be different. I went prepared. My flight was at 2 p.m. so I took a nice long run that morning and got in a quick weight workout. I packed two bananas and a plastic bag full of unsalted almonds and cashews. I took a commuter flight to Washington, DC, and had a 2-hour wait before my flight to Johannesburg, so I grabbed a meal—a hot turkey sandwich, mashed potatoes, some fruit, and a bottle of water. That filled me up so I wouldn't be hungry for the meal on the plane, which I planned on skipping. Plus, the mashed potatoes have a sedating effect. And I planned to get some sleep. Waiting for the plane to take off, I ate a banana—more calming carbs, man. Bananas are sleeping pills in a peel to me. Fully loaded with a belly full of sleepy-food, I didn't have to stay up for the flight meal. And I could take advantage of yet another sleep inducer: the G-forces on my body at takeoff. Ever notice how you become drowsy as your plane races down the runway? That's due to the Gs and the decreased oxygen in the cabin at takeoff. I slept for 9 hours on that flight—in coach! I arrived in Cape Town after the short flight from Johannesburg without suffering from jet lag, all because I planned and ate right.

PLAN AHEAD

Preparation is the key to keeping business trips from derailing your fitness—even if you're only traveling from New York to Boston. Use these tips to make your travel an opportunity to leave some extra baggage behind.

Drink water on the way to the airport. Then sip some more after you make it through check-in. Flying can dehydrate you easily. And cravings and hunger are often nothing more than an indication that you are thirsty, not hungry. Have a cup of water or juice about once every hour that you're in the air.

Stay out of the executive lounge. Don't tempt yourself with the free drinks and salted snacks offered in those hidden havens to which your platinum card gains you access. Instead, pack low-fat cheese sticks, baby carrots, hard-boiled eggs, bags of Cheerios and raisins, fruit, and slices of ham or turkey to eat while waiting for your flight.

Pack your own peanuts. Better yet, make them unsalted raw almonds. Rich in protein. They'll fill you up. Won't make you thirsty.

Bring a crossword puzzle. We snack when we're bored. Keep your mind and hands occupied during the flight.

Carry running shoes and shorts on board. Always have an extra set of workout gear packed in your carry-on bag so you don't have to think twice about it if you have to get on a plane at the spur of the moment.

Go for a run when you arrive. The best way to reset your internal clock on an overnight flight is to get out into the sunshine as soon as you arrive. If it's too early for check-in, drop your bags at the hotel, change into running gear in the hotel gym, and hit the pavement. Exercise is a terrific way to wake up and improve your mood, and running is a great opportunity to soak up some local color while soaking in some natural light. Ask the concierge to map out a good running route so you won't get lost.

Find a great gym. Most hotel fitness centers are nothing more than a guest room with two treadmills where the beds used to be. And one of the machines is usually out of order. Indeed, 55 percent of business travelers are so disappointed with hotel fitness facilities that these gyms actually become obstacles to staying in shape, according to a survey by Lieberman Research Worldwide. Don't risk it. Find a good health club before you leave and book some time there. For starters, check out www.menshealth.com/bestgyms/index.html for a list of the 30 best gyms in America. Or . . .

Hire a local trainer. If you need a little extra motivation, hire a personal trainer for an hour or two. Go to nsca-lift.org and use the "Find a Trainer" tool to locate a trainer near your destination. (It lists trainers abroad, too.) A trainer can get you into a good gym and build a workout that fits your needs. And the money you just spent will motivate you to show up for the workout.

Use your body weight. Don't forget to use your Belly Off! 2-Minute Drill on your trip. Do a 3-set circuit for a heart-pumping workout. Run the hotel's exit stairwell as well. You'll have it all to yourself. Pack resistance bands in your suitcase. Loop the band around a doorknob or wedge the strap on top of the door for lat pulldowns, curls, presses, and dozens of other exercises.

FIT FACT

100

Calories you'll save if you make a gin and tonic with seltzer as the mixer instead of tonic

Schedule some regional cross-training. If you're traveling to Long Beach, take a surfing lesson; in Colorado, ski or snowshoe; and in Vermont, hike, mountain bike, or kayak. Your hotel concierge can prearrange these activities to match your schedule. While the fresh air will do your body good, participating in the local sport will give you something besides business to chat with your client about over dinner. In fact, why not invite him or her along? Most locals never take advantage of what's right in their backyards.

Lose the key to the minibar. The hotel room minibar is a ridiculously expensive way to gain pounds. When you arrive at the hotel, refuse the minibar key. Or ask that the minibar be removed from your room. If you stare at that $12 bar of Toblerone long enough, you're going to devour it.

Make a new friend. Prescheduling a fitness date is one of the best ways to guarantee that you won't stop exercising on the road. If you need someone to play tennis against on your visit to San Francisco (or just about anywhere else in the world), find one through www.tennisrendezvous.com. Looking to get in 18 holes on your trip to Milwaukee? Try one of these online services to match you with other golfers according to your handicap: www.golfpartners.com; www.matchpractice.com; or www.mygolfbuddy.com. Sign up for a local 5-K on your next business trip by using *Runner's World* magazine's "racefinder" search tool at www.runnersworld.com.

Carry a thermos. It can be tough to find a whey protein shake when you're driving through Albuquerque. So, carry a sleek thermos bottle with you and Ziploc bags of premeasured powdered protein. You can always find milk or water. Shake it up for a quick meal replacement or a snack. To avoid the unmixed powder globules, pack the Ontel Personal Power Mixer, a battery-operated portable blender that doubles as a drinking glass, from www.ontelcatalog.com ($10).

SUPERSHOT
Take It Slow

Get a better workout on the elliptical machine or stairclimber by avoiding beginner mistakes. A lot of people use such little resistance and go so fast on the elliptical that their momentum propels their steps. Be sure to set the resistance so that you feel that you're pushing the ramp down with each step. On the stairclimber, avoid locking your elbows with your hands on the railing. That's like using crutches.

SURVIVE THE BUFFET

Your toughest obstacle on any business trip is the Trade Show Cocktail Party Buffet because it is just so abundant with delicious morsels, fried and sauce-laden. And it's free, which makes it even more tempting. Here are some tricks to keep you from blowing your good intentions to smithereens one lard-filled latke at a time.

Eat before you eat. Don't go to the party on an empty stomach. An hour before you leave, have a bowl of instant oatmeal or a banana, something to keep you from making a beeline to the buffet.

Drink a glass of tomato juice. The pulpy liquid has bulk to it and it will give your stomach some volume to take the edge off your appetite.

Navigate the buffet trays. Follow this order: Eat from the vegetable tray first. The high-water-volume, high-fiber fare will fill you up without delivering a lot of calories. Not full? Try shrimp and other seafood; then move on to grilled chicken or other lean meats. Pass by the breads, chips, sauce-laden pastas, and anything fried.

Take a dessert plate. Studies show that the more food options you have, the more you'll tend to sample. One study in the *Journal of Consumer Research* found that when a variety of foods are offered, such as at a buffet, people eat 43 percent more food. Use forced portion control to counter that tendency. Instead of grabbing the large entrée plate, use the dessert or salad plate and place only two items on it at a time. That'll encourage you to eat less and slow down your eating to allow time for feelings of stomach satiety to signal your brain that you are full.

Schmooze more. Focus on the social networking aspect of the party rather than the eating. Set a goal to talk to seven people who can help your career. If you have a mission you'll be less likely to munch mindlessly.

Practice stealth drinking. Drink a glass of ice water between beers and cocktails. It'll effectively cut your alcohol and calorie intake in half. Or fake it. Order a diet ginger ale in a scotch glass with a lemon. No one will know you're not drinking booze with the boys.

EATING ON THE ROAD

When you can't prepare your own meals, you give up a lot of control to the restaurant that serves you. So the best thing you can do is control massive portion sizes by leaving food on your plate. Asking the waiter to put half of your meal in a doggy bag before you even begin eating is a good strategy when you are going home to your own bed, but if you're heading back to a hotel, that's not practical. Instead, draw an imaginary line down the center of your plate and remind yourself to eat just half of your meal. We throw nutrition to the wind and ignore portion size when we travel on business. You need to fight that part of our human nature. Here are some other general tips, plus some smart meal choices to help you eat reasonably on the road.

Drink before you eat. Make sure you drink lots of water during the day. It'll make you feel fuller so you won't eat as much. Don't wait until mealtime to do this because fluids dilute digestive enzymes and can hamper absorption of vital nutrients, which are key to efficient energy metabolism. To curb your appetite before the big meal, guzzle 1 or 2 cups of water 30 minutes before dining out.

Have an appetizer an hour before dinner. Prep for a business dinner the way you would for that trade show buffet: Eat something about an hour before you leave so you aren't ravenous when you arrive at the restaurant. Then, when ordering, always choose a starter of soup (minestrone, gazpacho, or anything chicken-broth-based) or a salad. Both options are low glycemic (i.e., digested slowly), so they won't spike blood sugar levels, which, in turn, can trigger food cravings and feelings of hunger.

Eat in a clean, well-lighted place. Stay out of dark steak houses. Researchers at the University of Cali-

FAT FACT
When buying chips, choose single-serving sizes. A University of Illinois study found that buying larger package sizes leads to a 22 percent increase in calories consumed—regardless of how hungry you are.

fornia, Irvine, found that low lights increase binge eating. Dimmer lights make you less self-aware, which loosens your inhibitions, say the researchers.

Order dessert. Go ahead and have something sweet for a treat, but limit yourself to three bites. If you can't do that, don't have dessert.

WHAT TO EAT

BREAKFAST

This is the easiest meal to manage healthfully because the food choices at a diner or a hotel breakfast buffet are so similar to what you're eating at home. Give yourself enough time before your first meetings to eat a big breakfast. It'll start you on the right track for the day.

Avoid high-carbohydrate options like the pancakes, French toast, waffles, bagels and muffins (usually made from white flour), and home fries (the breakfast equivalent of french fries). Instead, start out with a fiber-packed bowl of oatmeal sweetened with a handful of raisins. Order a spinach and feta cheese omelet, one of the most nutritious choices on the menu. (Feta cheese has about a third less fat than Cheddar.) Ask for half an omelet. Most hotel restaurants and diners make them the size of a Frisbee. Instead of sausage or regular bacon, choose Canadian bacon; it's higher in protein than ham and lower in fat, just about 2 grams per slice. Toast? Whole-wheat, of course.

LUNCH

You can't go wrong with most vegetable salads for lunch if you control the dressings. But what if the lunch spot is a burger joint, pizzeria, or a Mexican or Chinese restaurant? Build a healthier eating game plan for each occasion and order the same thing religiously every time you go to one of these spots so you won't be tempted by bad choices.

At the burger joint: Forget about the fries, of course. You're better off ordering two regular burgers, dumping one bun and making a double-decker. Hold the mayo. If you're eating at McDonald's or Burger King, choose the regular hamburger or a Whopper Jr. instead of those fried fish fillet sandwiches. You'll save lots of calories and grams of fat.

At the pizza place: Start out with a small garden salad and a glass of water to fill you up. And limit yourself to one pizza slice by reminding yourself that each one packs about 300 calories and 11 grams of fat. If you must have two slices, try to make one a pizza marinara, which doesn't have cheese but does have a lot of vitamin-rich tomato sauce. Skip the soda. Order an unsweetened iced tea or flavored water.

At the taco spot: First, ask the waiter to remove the basket of tortilla chips. They are loaded with fat. Soft tortillas are generally lower in fat than hard-shell tortillas, so go for one burrito. A chicken burrito is a good choice. A bean burrito is even better, due to the fiber and protein, unless it's made with refried beans, which are typically cooked in lard. Ask about the beans. If they offer black or red beans—*ole!* Another good option is the fajitas. Just eat the meat, peppers, and onions and avoid the flour tortillas, which are heavy in calories and carbs. You usually get a side of black or red beans with it. And order some guacamole. Made from avocados, it's rich in heart-healthy monounsaturated fats, and it delivers a good dose of vitamin E.

At the Chinese restaurant: Start with egg-drop or hot-and-sour soup to tame your hunger. Almost every Chinese restaurant offers a "Vegetarian's Delight," typically made up of steamed vegetables over a scoop of steamed rice. Ask for brown rice instead of white to get more fiber. Avoid the egg rolls and anything breaded or deep-fried or covered with that gooey, sugary brown sauce or sweet-and-sour sauce. Use chopsticks instead of a fork. You'll eat more slowly and may end up eating less.

SUPERSHOT
Put Down
Your Fork

After taking a bite, place your fork on the table. Talk to your neighbor. Anything you can do to slow down your eating will help you save calories. A recent study at the University of Rhode Island found that fast eaters consumed about 67 more calories per meal than people who took their time. Here's why: It takes a little time (maybe as much as 20 minutes) for feelings of satiety to register in your brain.

DINNER

Here's where your habit of snacking healthfully throughout the day can pay off. Let your clients order the fried calamari appetizer and the béarnaise sauce for their steak. Having arrived at the restaurant without hunger pangs, you'll be a model of self-discipline. Later that night, you'll sleep more soundly without having a typical expense-account meal sitting in your gut. And chances are you won't drip melted butter on your tie.

At the steak house: Grilled salmon is always an excellent choice, but if you want beef, go for the grilled top-round steak or petit filet. Both are less fatty than the perennial biz-dinner favorite, the rib eye. Ask for an extra serving of steamed vegetables instead of the baked potatoes. Or see if they can get you a baked sweet potato, which packs more fiber and vitamins than a spud does. Some steak houses offer game meats. Consider trying them. Cornish game hen, venison, ostrich, and bison are all quite lean. Start with a soup or salad to keep hunger at bay.

ROAD RULES
Maintenance Tips for Business and Pleasure Trips

1. Drink 1 cup of water per hour on the plane to avoid dehydration. (Orange juice, tea, seltzer, or tomato juices are good substitutes for water to mix things up, but stay away from beer, wine, and liquor.)

2. Walk the aisle every 90 minutes during the flight to stretch your legs.

3. Buy snacks for the airport and flight—there will be delays. Good choices: Au Bon Pain salads and/or fruit-yogurt parfait; Nature Valley Crunchy Granola Bars.

4. Try to maintain your regular sleep schedule and get 7 to 8 hours per night.

5. If you're driving a car for your business trip, pack a Ziploc bag full of dried fruit and nuts. You'll be less likely to swing through the drive-thru at the first hunger pang. Dried fruit is driver-friendly: There's nothing to peel or drip down your sleeve. Nuts like cashews and almonds will fill you up and provide a protein boost.

6. Call ahead to your hotel and ask them to have a salad, fruit, yogurt, an omelet, or hard-boiled eggs waiting for you upon arrival.

7. Buy an apple or an orange to keep in your room for the morning.

8. If you're grabbing coffee at Starbucks, avoid any drink that requires flavorings, including anything with "mocha" or "caramel" in their names. You'll save up to 100 calories.

9. Work out in the morning before you fly, if possible. Take a walk when you get to your destination if time allows, especially if it is daylight.

10. Don't eat a main meal after 8 p.m.

At the Italian restaurant: Start with antipasto for the protein. Then have a bowl of minestrone soup. The fiber-rich beans and vegetables will fill you up. One of the best entrée choices is a slice of lasagna, provided it's not the size of the Roman Coliseum. If it is, eat half. Usually made with lower-in-fat ricotta cheese, it'll generally pack fewer calories than, say, any parmigiana dish, which is typically breaded, fried, and smothered with mozzarella cheese. And it delivers a reasonable balance of protein, fat, and carbohydrate. Nibble on one or two of those thin packaged bread sticks versus the basket of garlic bread.

At the seafood restaurant: Easy to be good here, right? Yes, if you stay away from: tartar sauce, which packs 10 grams of fat in a single tablespoon; fried crab cakes, fried shrimp, fried oysters, fried flounder (see a pattern?); New England clam chowder (made with cream); and hush puppies (deep-fried cornmeal). Eat instead grilled salmon, tuna, bluefish, striped bass, almost anything grilled or broiled (but watch the butter). Start with an appetizer of shrimp cocktail with cocktail sauce, which is virtually fat-free. Tomato-based Manhattan-style clam chowder or fish stews made with light broths are good starter choices, too. Always choose steamed vegetables and rice over french fries.

At the Indian restaurant: At the risk of sounding repetitive, start your meal with a soup. Most Indian soups are packed with vegetables. Next, check the menu for vegetable curries made with dal, stewed black lentils which are a terrific source of low-fat protein and fiber. Also look for dishes based on chickpeas, spinach, tomatoes, and mushrooms. Tandoori chicken, fish, or shrimp is a terrific choice because it's baked in a clay oven. Shy away from the fried foods and the lamb, traditionally made from the fattiest cuts of meat. Naan? This charred flatbread is delicious. Be careful about overindulging.

SUPERSHOT
Put 'Er in Reverse

When unmotivated to workout, try reversing the order in which you do your exercises. Sports psychologists say this simple trick can provide the mental boost you need to keep exercising.

REAL GUYS—REAL RESULTS

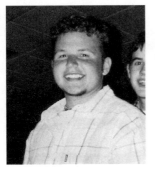

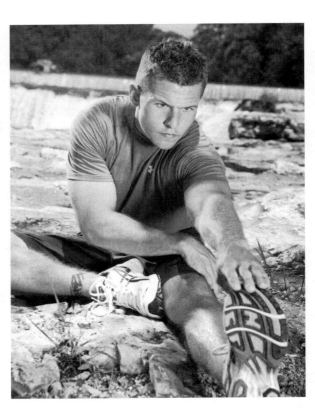

BEFORE:
253
POUNDS

AFTER:
169
POUNDS

"A New Year's Resolution Saved My Life."

VITALS: **Erik Bartlett, 22, Joplin, MO**
OCCUPATION: **Student**
HEIGHT: **5'10"**
LESSON LEARNED: **Exercise is a lifelong change, not just a temporary solution.**

Bartlett played sports as a kid until video games became his life in high school. He would sometimes drink eight sodas and eat a whole bag of chips while playing.

THE TURNING POINT

On New Year's Day in 2004, he resolved to get in shape. A friend of his helped him design a rigorous fitness plan: 45 minutes on the elliptical trainer twice a day, 5 days a week. He overhauled his diet with chicken, egg whites, and fruit, and he cut out fast food and pizza. In 3 months he lost 50 pounds. But that was just the beginning.

LIFE IN THE FIT LANE

Bartlett's routine now consists of hour-long cardio sessions 4 days a week, plus an hour of weight lifting every day. "I eat about six small meals a day to keep my body fueled for exercise," says Bartlett.

THE REWARD

"It's nice to hear compliments and congratulations from people who haven't seen me in a while," he says. Bartlett also gains satisfaction from training for an upcoming marathon and adventure race.

BARTLETT'S BEST BELLY OFF! TIPS:

• Make sacrifices. Instead of going out with friends, go to the gym.
• Break up your cardio. If you can't fit in an hour on the treadmill, break up the workout into a longer session before work in the morning and shorter, less-intense sessions later on.
• Stay focused. Just because it's the weekend doesn't mean you get a free pass to slack off on eating right and exercising.
• Don't feel guilty. On days when you miss a workout or eat too much, chalk it up to being human. Give yourself a break.
• Keep a photograph of yourself at your heaviest weight, for motivation.

13

BELLY OFF! MAINTENANCE AND MOTIVATION

How to Stay Lean for Life

CONGRATULATIONS. By now you've slimmed down and dramatically improved your fitness and your health. Go ahead and toast yourself with a frosty cold lager or something else you've been craving. MoonPies? Sure. You deserve it.

Now comes the tricky part: keeping the weight off for good. You'll gain it back if you go back to your old ways. Fortunately, you've learned a thing or two about how your body responds to food, and you've made exercise a regular part of your lifestyle. That muscle you've added helps fry calories even when you're sitting around on the couch watching Giada lick gelato on the Food Network.

FAT FACT

Being overweight quadruples your risk of back injury.

Of course, there's always the danger of slipping back to belly central. A new job might saddle you with tons of work. A new baby might keep you up all night. A twisted knee might keep you off the treadmill. All three of those things happened to me a couple of years back. But the meniscus tear in my left knee gave me the easiest excuse to stop running, which led to a lot of sitting around with my face in a bag of Chips Ahoy! cookies. I had arthroscopic surgery to clip the shredded cartilage, and although my doctor told me to stretch and go to rehab, I babied my knee for 4 weeks, which allowed me to lose my fitness momentum.

If I stop exercising, I tend to get lazy in other parts of my life, especially my diet. And that's what happened after my surgery. I started eating more junk food. When baby Sophia would wake Kathy and me in the middle of the night for a feeding, I'd sneak down to the fridge for a snack or a glass of ginger ale. I ate more of my lunches at my desk at work and found that I was snacking more there, too. In a very short period, I had joined the ranks of the 80 percent of exercisers and dieters who fall off their well-intended programs.

My point is that setbacks are common, and it's likely that you will struggle at times with finding the motivation to maintain the gains (and losses!) you've made on the Belly Off! Diet. At times like these, spending time online with the other members of the Belly Off! Club at www.menshealth.com/bellyoff can really pay off. And you can always go back to your 7-Day Quick-Start in Chapter 4 and recommit to the principles of the program:

- Spark your metabolism every morning with the Belly Off! 2-Minute Drill and a nutritious, protein-rich breakfast.

- Eat small meals four to six times a day—to stifle cravings and bingeing.

- Exercise with your bodyweight or barbells and do interval training.

- Avoid cakes, cookies, and other processed foods while eating fiber-rich, nutrient-dense whole grains, vegetables, and fruits, plus protein.

- Limit your consumption of liquid calories, especially alcohol. (Congratulations, you can have beer again! But keep consumption to three or four alcoholic beverages per week. Remember, the carbs and alcohol in beer, wine, and Alabama slammers act like liquid fat and that fat will home right in on your belly.)

Meanwhile, here are some motivational tips and tricks that we've collected from trainers, exercise physiologists, psychologists, and Belly Off! Club members over the years that may help you to . . .

STICK WITH IT

Use Visual Cues. Remember that "before" photograph you took of yourself prior to starting the Belly Off! program? Hang it in a place where you'll see it every day. Now tape a photo of your new, thinner self next to the fat photo. There's visual motivation for you. Before and ever after. Share your success story with the world by posting your photos and story at www.menshealth.com/bellyoff. Nothing firms up a commitment like going public.

Weigh yourself every day. It'll remind you of your goals and provide you with positive feedback. Remember what you learned in Chapter 1. People who weighed themselves every day were 82 percent more likely to keep their weight off than people who didn't use a scale, according to a recent study at the Weight Control and Diabetes Research Center in Providence, Rhode Island. For the most accurate readings, weigh yourself at the same time every day, since weight can fluctuate by several pounds at different times of the day.

Put money on your muscle. If you hired a personal trainer and cancelled a session without notice, you'd

FIT FACT
Exercise helps your brain stick to a diet by reinforcing your weight-loss goal and drive, according to a study at the University of Pittsburgh.

FAT FACT

86

Percentage of
Americans who
could be overweight
or obese by 2030 if
current trends
continue, according
to a report in the
journal *Obesity*

still have to pay the trainer. Treat yourself the same way. If you miss a workout, pay a spouse or friend $20. Or pay yourself, say, $20 for every good workout. Stash the money in a fund, and reward yourself when you reach a weight-loss goal. Here's an idea: Buy yourself some new clothes. You'll need them after losing all that weight!

Add workouts to your Outlook. Schedule your workouts on a calendar. And cross off each one completed with a black marker. Or plug workouts into your computer's Outlook calendar for reminder alerts. Researchers who tested this system found that exercisers who tracked their workouts were more successful at sticking with their plans than those who didn't.

Take a day off. Schedule a cheat day—mine is Sunday. That's when I rest and eat whatever I want. (Reese's Peanut Butter Cups.) It gives me a psychological boost. (Strombolis.) If on Tuesday I really want Oreos, I know I have to wait until Sunday. By then, either I don't crave them anymore, or I'll eat them and feel extra motivated for my workout on Monday. A cheat day is a technique used effectively for motivation and education by the trainers on NBC's *Biggest Loser* reality television show. One day every week at the Biggest Loser ranch is "high-calorie day" when contestants can go over their calorie limits. "We do it to make the point that eating healthy doesn't mean a life of deprivation," explains trainer Bob Harper. "You can't sustain that. You want to develop healthy habits that you can live with." The contestants typically order out for burritos. "The next day, they really feel the effects of all the sugar and sodium-filled food," says Harper. "They feel like crap. They learn very quickly that a healthy body that's been exercising and eating right doesn't want all that fat and processed junk."

Chart your progress. Just as weighing yourself provides motivation through daily feedback, keeping a workout log can motivate you by charting your progress. Just write the exercises on a sheet of paper and create three columns, one for each workout in the week. Give yourself enough room in each column to record the weight you use and the number of repetitions you perform in each set. Make a few dozen copies of that sheet, start a new one each week, and keep them all in chronological order in a binder. That way, you can quickly flip through and see your progress from one week to the next.

Eat a pickle. When a craving for something salty and crunchy threatens your good intentions, reach for a pickle instead of the Pringles. Dill spears, at just 1 calorie each, will cover both cravings.

Wake up at 6:25. If you find you're skipping breakfast, wake up 5 minutes earlier. Five minutes is all you need to toast some whole-wheat bread, heat instant oatmeal, or microwave some sausage links. Remember that eating breakfast will help you eat less later in the day.

Don't count calories. A good diet is effortless. By eating the right foods, you'll eliminate hunger and control your calorie intake automatically.

Take a hot shower. Some marathoners, football players, hockey players, and other athletes take a hot shower a few hours before starting a race or a competition. The hot water warms up muscles enough to loosen them for physical stress.

Bet on your success. In one study, people who bet that they could stick to a workout program for 6 months scored a 97 percent success rate. Wager with a workout partner—first guy to wimp out pays up.

Suck on an Altoid. Smelling peppermint can boost exercise performance. Researchers say that the scent of mint alters your perception of how hard you're exercising, which can make workouts seem less strenuous so you'll exercise longer.

Schedule an exercise meeting. When work gets so busy that you have trouble fitting in a workout, schedule a running meeting with your colleagues. It's a smart way to multitask. This strategy is actually pretty popular with the editors of *Men's Health* for brainstorming sessions. Some of our best ideas come

SUPERSHOT
Ride Higher,
Go Longer

Setting your saddle height on your bicycle so that your knees are bent at a 25-degree angle (from vertical) at the bottom of the pedal stroke may help you ride longer without fatiguing, according to a study from the University of Central Arkansas. Pedaling at this angle lets you use the least amount of energy for your work, say researchers. To find the proper saddle height for you, visit a local bike shop.

out of noontime jogs up the mountain near our Pennsylvania offices.

Crank Eddie Van Halen's "Eruption." Reams of research show that if you work out to your favorite music, you'll work out longer and more intensely. In one study involving women, those who exercised to music lost 8 pounds more than women who sweated in silence. What to listen to? Whatever you like, but make it fast paced. Researchers from the U.K. discovered that the faster the tune that you listen to, the more vigorously you'll push yourself.

Take that first step. No matter how tired you are, exercise will make you feel better. Taking those first few steps after a tough day at work is difficult, but research shows that working out raises your energy level and improves your mood.

Join a team. Don't underestimate the power of friends. The team camaraderie you get from playing organized sports is terrific motivation, says Belly Off! Club member Josh Samara, of Oklahoma City.

Change your pace. Every 3 weeks, try a different weight workout. Every new season, choose a different cross-training activity or sport. Heck, make it a game. FitDeck is a deck of 50 playing cards, each with a different exercise on it, from abs to arms to full-body movements. Shuffle it and select 10 or 20 cards for your workout. Flip each card over one by one, follow the instructions, and go for it. You can even play in teams. The deck is $19 at www.fitdeck.com.

BOOK COURT TIME FOR 2015

The biggest lesson to learn through any diet and exercise program is that the program doesn't end once you reach your weight-loss goal. There's no finish line. It is simply your new lifestyle. Every day for the rest of your life you will make better food choices and move your body around. The Belly Off! Diet is designed to build a foundation of habits for you to fall back on no matter what comes down the pike 3 months or 5 years from now.

REAL GUYS—REAL RESULTS

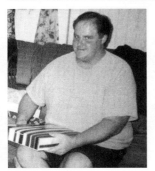

BEFORE:
374
POUNDS

AFTER:
192
POUNDS

"I've added years back to my life."

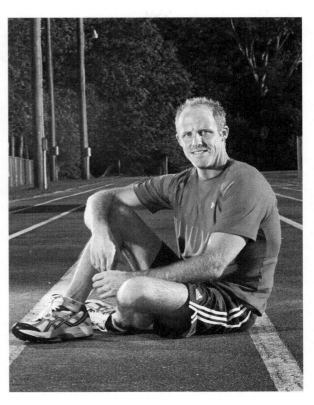

VITALS: **Brandon Watford, 30, Bonifay, FL**
OCCUPATION: **Salesman**
HEIGHT: **6'2"**
LESSON LEARNED: **Set small goals. Trying to drop big numbers can seem impossible at first.**

Brandon Watford was chubby all of his young life. "My mom told me it was baby fat, but it never went away," says Watford. His love of traditional Southern fare—fried chicken, sweet iced tea, and biscuits with gravy—didn't help. By his early 20s, climbing a few steps winded him, and his self-esteem had evaporated. "Eventually, all I wanted to do was sleep all day," he says.

THE TURNING POINT

At 24, Watford weighed 374 pounds and his total cholesterol topped 300. His doctor recommended a gastric bypass, but Watford resisted. "I realized I could make the lifestyle changes that were needed for me to lose weight on my own," he says. He eliminated bread and deep-fried foods and walked 2 hours on the treadmill every day.

LIFE IN THE FIT LANE

Watford now walks 5 miles a day and lifts weights 4 days a week. He chugs water constantly and typically eats oatmeal for breakfast, a salad for lunch, and baked chicken for dinner. "It's all about balance. If I eat a big lunch, then I eat a smaller dinner."

THE REWARD

By nearly cutting his weight in half, Watford has regained his confidence and energy. And his health has turned a corner. He no longer needs his blood pressure medicines, and his cholesterol numbers have dropped to a healthy level. "I've added years back to my life," he says.

WATFORD'S BEST BELLY-OFF! TIPS

●Lift as you lose. Lifting even light weights helps tighten loose skin.
●Change it up. If you plateau on the scale, alter your diet to nudge your body back into weight-loss mode.
●Discover new cuisines. There are dozens of ways to cook chicken, and most are healthier than frying.

APPENDIX

UNDERSTANDING GLYCEMIC LOAD
A Guide to Help You Keep Blood Sugar in Check

The glycemic load is a system designed to rate a food's effect on your body's biochemistry, specifically your blood sugar and insulin levels. It's more useful than simply knowing the amount of carbohydrates in a food, because it differentiates between types of carbs, which can affect your body in different ways. For example, the body breaks down glucose in a potato much more rapidly than it breaks down pure sugar, spiking glucose levels in the blood and increasing the risk of diabetes.

In general, the lower a food's glycemic load value the better.
Low GL = 10 or lower
Medium GL = 11 to 19
High GL = 20 or higher

The glycemic load chart is a useful general guide to help you identify foods that will spike your blood sugar. But just as we don't think you should go through life counting every calorie, we don't recommend memorizing glycemic load. When trying to lose weight, it's much easier to simply stay away from sugary foods like cookies, cakes, juices, and sodas and limit starchy foods like white bread, white rice, pasta, and potatoes. By increasing your consumption of lean protein and nonstarchy vegetables and fruits, you'll automatically limit your intake of high-glycemic-load foods.

	GLYCEMIC LOAD PER SERVING
Baked Goods and Breakfast Breads	
Flan caramel custard	51
Pancakes	39
Corn muffin	30
French baguette with butter and strawberry jam	26
Bagel	25
Vanilla cake with vanilla frosting	24
Chocolate cake with chocolate frosting	20
Angel food cake	19
Banana cake made with sugar	18
Blueberry muffin	17
Croissant	17
Doughnut	17
Bran muffin	15
Apple pie made with sugar	13
Frozen waffles	10
Beans and Nuts	
Navy beans	12
Baked beans	7
Black beans	7
Kidney beans	7
Lentils	5
Cashews	3
Peanuts	1
Beverages	
Cranberry juice cocktail	24
Carrot juice	23
Orange soda	23
Coca-Cola	16
Apple juice, unsweetened	13
Orange juice, unsweetened	13
Chocolate milk	12
Gatorade	12

	GLYCEMIC LOAD PER SERVING
Hot chocolate	11
Tomato juice, unsweetened	4
Breads	
French baguette	15
Corn tortilla	12
Kaiser roll	12
White bread	10
Pita bread, white	10
Hamburger bun	9
Oat-bran bread	9
Whole-wheat tortilla	8
Whole-wheat bread	7
Spelt multigrain bread	7
Pumpernickel bread	5
Breakfast Cereals	
Instant Cream of Wheat	22
Cornflakes	21
Corn Pops	21
Cocoa Krispies	20
Instant oatmeal	17
Muesli	16
Cheerios	15
Shredded wheat	15
Oatmeal	13
Raisin Bran	12
All-Bran	4
Cookies and Crackers	
Rice cakes	17
Graham crackers	14
Vanilla wafers	14
Saltine crackers	12
Soda crackers	12
Stoned Wheat Thins	12

(continued)

	GLYCEMIC LOAD PER SERVING
Cookies and Crackers (cont.)	
Rye crispbread	10
Shortbread	10
Dairy Products	
Ice cream	8
Low-fat yogurt with fruit	7
Milk, fat-free	4
Milk, whole	3
Low-fat yogurt, artificially sweetened	2
Fruit	
Dates, dried	42
Raisins	28
Banana	13
Peach, canned in light syrup	9
Grapes	8
Apple	6
Orange	5
Peach	5
Pear	4
Watermelon	4
Cherries	3
Grapefruit	3
Pasta and Noodles	
Macaroni and cheese	32
Spaghetti, white	27
Macaroni	23
Fettuccini	18
Spaghetti, whole-wheat	16
Cheese tortellini	11
Snack Foods	
Skittles	32
Mars bar	27
Fruit Roll-Up	24
Jelly beans	22
Snickers bar	19

	GLYCEMIC LOAD PER SERVING
Doritos	18
Corn chips	17
Twix cookie bar	17
Pretzels, baked	16
Potato chips	11
Microwave popcorn	8
Nutella	4
Soup	
Black bean soup	17
Split pea soup	16
Lentil soup	9
Minestrone soup	7
Rice and Grains	
Instant white rice	29
Couscous	23
White rice	23
Sweet corn on the cob	17
Bulgur wheat	12
Pearled barley	11
Vegetables	
Baked russet potato	26
Instant mashed potatoes	17
Sweet potato	17
Boiled white potatoes	14
Yam	13
Parsnips	12
Carrots	3
Green peas	3
Miscellaneous	
French fries	22
Pizza with cheese	22
Honey	10
Chicken nuggets, microwaveable	7
Hummus (mashed chickpea dip)	0

INDEX

Boldface page references indicate photographs. <u>Underscored</u> references indicate boxed text and charts.

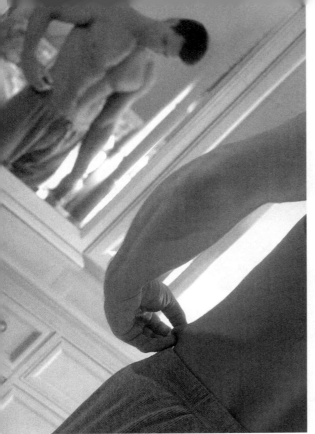

Don't just look in the mirror, look GOOD in the mirror.

Replace flab with lean, strong muscle in no time— with *THE BELLY OFF! DIET.*™

JOIN THE CLUB THAT'S LOST 1,836,987 POUNDS—AND COUNTING!

The Belly Off! Diet is based on the real-world examples of more than 80 men whose stories have been chronicled in the "Belly Off!" column in *Men's Health* magazine over the past 8 years, plus the weight loss strategies of some of the 300,000 other men who've signed up for the **Men's Health Belly Off! Club**. All told, these men have lost nearly 2 million pounds.

Following the Belly Off! Diet, you will:

■ Lose fat and shape up fast with the 7-Day Quick-Start Plan!

■ Add lean, strong muscle with the Bodyweight 100!

■ Drop inches off your waist while eating real food—including pizza, steak, and burgers!

■ Discover how to trigger your cells to burn belly fat first!

■ Learn the six core strategies that have helped our guys lose weight and keep it off!

Get your copy and join the online program at

BELLYOFF.COM/LOSEFAT

201075501